Noncardiac Chest Pain

A Growing Medical Problem

Noncardiac Chest Pain

A Growing Medical Problem

Ronnie Fass, MD
Guy D. Eslick, PhD

Editors

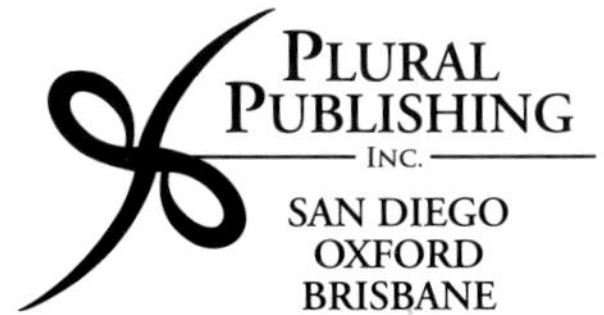

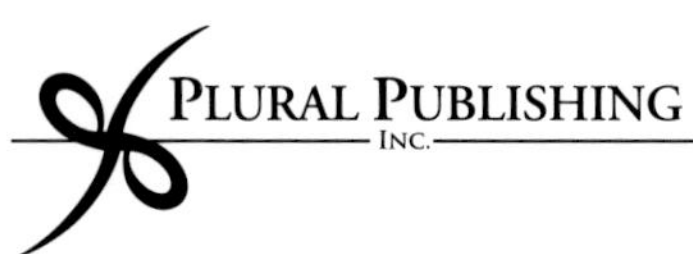

5521 Ruffin Road
San Diego, CA 92123

e-mail: info@pluralpublishing.com
Web site: http://www.pluralpublishing.com

49 Bath Street
Abingdon, Oxfordshire OX14 1EA
United Kingdom

Library of Congress Cataloging-in-Publication Data:

Noncardiac chest pain : a growing medical problem / [edited by] Ronnie Fass,
  Guy D. Eslick.
        p. ; cm.
   Includes bibliographical references.
   ISBN-13: 978-1-59756-176-1 (hardcover)
   ISBN-10: 1-59756-176-2 (hardcover)
   1. Chest pain. 2.   Chest pain—Etiology. 3.   Diagnosis, Differential. I.
 Fass, Ronnie. II. Eslick, Guy D.
   [DNLM: 1.   Chest Pain—diagnosis. 2.   Chest Pain—etiology. 3.   Chest
 Pain—therapy. WF 970 N812 2007]
   RC941.N6682 2007
   617.5'4—dc22
                                                          2007004292

Contents

Preface

"... the breast is often the seat of pains which are distressing sometimes even from their vehemence, oftener from their duration, as they have continued to tease the patient for six, for eight, for nine, and for 14 years. There have been several examples of their returning periodically every night ... There has appeared no reason to judge that they proceed from any cause of much importance to health ... or that they lead to any dangerous consequences."

William Heberden (1802)

Noncardiac chest pain (NCCP) remains an enigmatic condition that continues to represent a major challenge not only to modern gastroenterology, but also the fields of cardiology and psychiatric medicine. It is a poorly understood and heterogeneous condition with numerous underlying potential mechanisms. Limited progress has been made in recent years; however, there is a dearth of good quality clinical studies, pathophysiological research as well as population and hospital epidemiological data. Noncardiac chest pain is a very common and debilitating condition which impacts greatly on individual's both physically and psychosocially. The most complex and difficult aspects of noncardiac chest pain remain its diagnosis and management.

For the first time, there is a book that provides a comprehensive review of noncardiac chest pain. We have gathered the current world authorities in the field who have provided their insights and expertise on a variety of topics including epidemiology, cardiologist's perspective, pathophysiology, nonesophageal causes, sensory testing, psychological disorders, diagnosis, use of proton-pump inhibitors, brain imaging, economics, treatment, quality of life, prognosis and future developments.

We hope that this book provides not only current and useful information but also encouragement to physicians and researchers, leading to a greater interest in noncardiac chest pain from both a clinical and research perspective.

Ronnie Fass
Arizona, U.S.A.
Guy D. Eslick
Sydney, Australia
2007

Contributors

Sami R. Achem, MD, FACP, FACG, AGAF
Professor of Medicine
Mayo College of Medicine
Mayo Clinic
Jacksonville, Florida
Chapter 4

Qasim Aziz, PhD, GRCP
Professor of Gastroenerology
Dept of GI Sciences
University of Manchester
Hope Hospital
Manchester, United Kingdom
Chapter 5 and 9

Kenneth R. DeVault, MD, FACG
Professor of Medicine
Mayo Clinic College of Medicine
Jacksonville, Florida
Chapter 4

Guy D. Eslick, PhD, MMedSc (Clin Epi), MMedStat.
Clinical Epidemiologist
Department of Medicine
University of Sydney
Nepean Hospital
Penrith, New South Wales
Australia
Chapters 1, 6, 11-13

Ronnie Fass MD, FACP, FACG
Professor of Medicine
School of Medicine

University of Arizona
Head, Neuroenteric Clinical Research
  Group
Director GI Motility Laboratories
Southern Arizona VA Health Care
  System and
University of Arizona Health Sciences
  Center
Tucson Arizona
Chapters 3, 7, 8, 10, 14

Elisa M. Faybush, MD
Private Practice
Mesa, Arizona
Chapter 7

Paul E. Fenster, MD, FACC
Associate Professor of Medicine
Section of Cardiology
University of Arizona, Saver Heart
  Center
Tucson, Arizona
Chapter 2

Anthony R. Hobson, PhD
Clinical Scientist
GI Discovery Medicine
Neurology & Gi CEDD
GSK R&D Limited
Chapter 9

Jae Geun Hyun, MD
Gastroenterology Fellow
The Mount Sinai Medical Center
New York, New York
Chapter 3

Anmarie Easley Moore, MD
Fellow in Gastroenterology
Department of Medicine
Division of Gastroenterology
University of Arizona
Tucson, Arizona
Chapter 10

Justin L. Sewell, MD, MPH
Resident Physician, Internal Medicine
University of California, San Francisco
San Francisco, California
Chapter 3

Michael Shapiro, MD
Research Fellow
The Neuroenteric Clinical Research
  Group
Southern Arizona VA Health Care
  system
University of Arizona Health Sciences
  Center
Tucson, Arizona
Chapter 10

Abhishek Sharma, MBChB, MRCP
Clinical Research Fellow
Department of GI Sciences
University of Manchester
Hope Hospital
Manchester, UK
Chapter 5

**Vincent L. Sorrell, MD, FACC, FACP,
FASE**
Associate Professor of Clinical Medicine
  and Radiology
Allan C. Hudson and Helen Lovaas
  Chair of Cardiac Imaging
Departments of Medicine and Radiology
University of Arizona, Sarver Heart Center
Tucson, Arizona
Chapter 2

**Wai-Man Wong, MD, PhD, FACP,
FACG, FRCP**
Honorary Clinical Associate Professor
Department of Medicine
University of Hong Kong, China
Chapter 8

*To my wife Shira and my children Ofer, Hagar, and Sharon
for your unconditional love and support.*

RF

To my wife Wilma

GE

CHAPTER 1

Epidemiology

Guy D. Eslick

History

Historically, ancient physicians made no accurate record or descriptions of chest pain in ancient or medieval times. There are conflicting reports as to who first provided an accurate description of chest pain.[1] Traditionally, the honor of the first published record of chest pain (angina pectoris) goes to Dr William Heberden, who presented his paper on how to take and record a medical history from an individual with chest pain at the Royal College of Physicians in London in 1768; the work was subsequently published in the College Journal in 1772 (Fig 1-1).[2]

Introduction

There is no question that William Heberden's report instigated an enormous interest in the potential pathology and consequences resulting from chest pain. There has been much research done on the clinical aspects of chest pain over the last two centuries, especially in relation to acute coronary syndromes, but chest pain of noncardiac origin remains poorly understood in many facets. This is particularly true in terms of the epidemiology and natural history of noncardiac chest pain (NCCP) which has been inadequately studied; the evidence of this lies in the dearth of adequately designed and powered epidemiologic studies to assess the natural history, prevalence/incidence, and outcomes of this condition.

Definition and Classification

Noncardiac chest pain is a very complex disorder and no standard definition exists. There are a few reasons why defining noncardiac chest pain is difficult; the major reason relates to the fact that there are so many different synonyms (currently there are around 20 different terms) used in the medical literature to describe this heterogeneous condition,

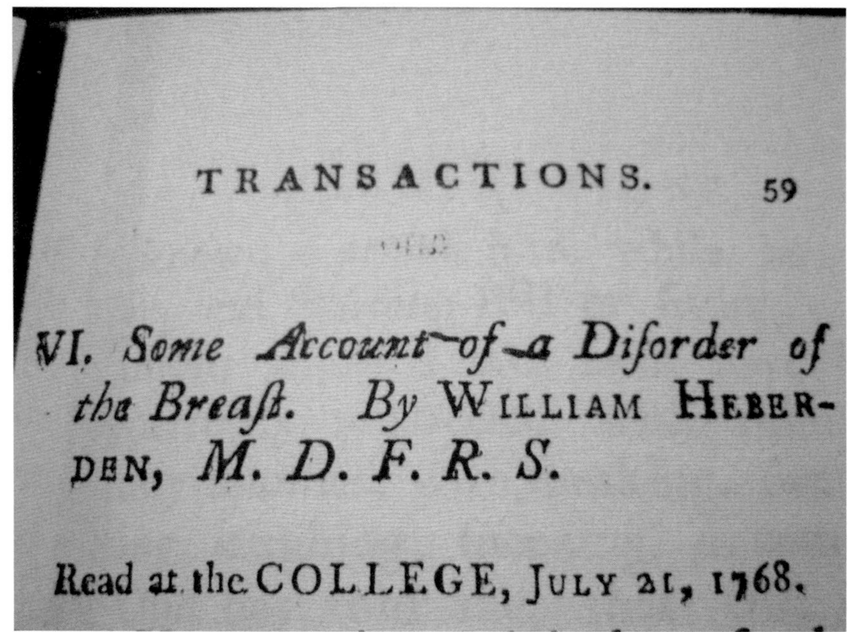

Fig 1–1. Opening page of the manuscript credited as the first record published of chest pain. (From Heberden W. Some account of a disorder of the breast. *Medical Transactions of the Royal College of Physicians of London.* 1772;2:59-67.)

there is substantial overlap in the terms used among different medical specialities. These terms usually fall into two groups: those that are all inclusive and those that target a specific subset of patients with chest pain. As the term "noncardiac" implies, it is essentially all chest pain that does not have a cardiac origin, making it an extremely long list of possible conditions.

The recently revised Rome III criteria for functional gastrointestinal disorders have modified the definition for functional chest pain of presumed esophageal origin to "episodes of unexplained chest pain that usually are midline in location and of visceral quality, and therefore potentially of esophageal origin. The pain is easily confused with cardiac angina and pain from other esophageal disorders, including achalasia and gastroesophageal reflux disease (GERD)."[3] The diagnostic

criteria for functional chest pain of presumed esophageal origin must include all of the following:

- Midline chest pain or discomfort that is not of burning quality
- Absence of evidence that gastroesophageal reflux is the cause of the symptom
- Absence of histopathology-based esophageal motility disorders

These criteria must be fulfilled for the last 3 months with symptom onset at least 6 months before diagnosis.

Using the Rome III criteria for defining functional chest pain may be useful in assisting in diagnosing patients; however, these criteria have never been reported in the medical literature as part of a research study or clinical report. The number of studies using the term "functional chest pain" is extremely small ($n = 16$) based on a MEDLINE search (1966–2006), with the majority of these not using the Rome criteria. However, a few published reports have used the Rome I and II criteria in assessing the epidemiology of functional chest pain.[4-6] Does the lack of reporting using these criteria mean that the criteria used are too specific, or is it just that "functional chest pain" is an inconsequential subset of noncardiac chest pain, or is "functional chest pain" the noncardiac chest pain? Additional future studies from around the world will be required to answer these questions.

A recent review article provided two commonly used definitions for noncardiac chest pain.[7] The first was "chest pain that is not angina (retrosternal pain precipitated by exertion and relieved by rest) and is not chest pain due to ischemic heart disease," and the second "recurrent episodes of substernal chest pain or discomfort that should be diagnosed only after excluding nonesophageal causes such as cardiac, musculoskeletal, pleuritic, pulmonary, and other disorders." These are obviously different definitions, but are either of them adequate for defining noncardiac chest pain? Currently, no definition appears adequate in classifying noncardiac chest pain.

Prevalence Studies

Community-Based Studies

There is a paucity of population-based studies which report on the epidemiology of noncardiac chest pain. Currently, worldwide there are only a handful of studies that have determined the population prevalence of noncardiac chest pain.[8-12] The lowest prevalence rates of noncardiac chest pain come from Hong Kong,[11] whereas Australia appears to have the highest prevalence,[8] with Europe[9,11] and the United States[10] having rates in between these two countries (Fig 1–2). It should

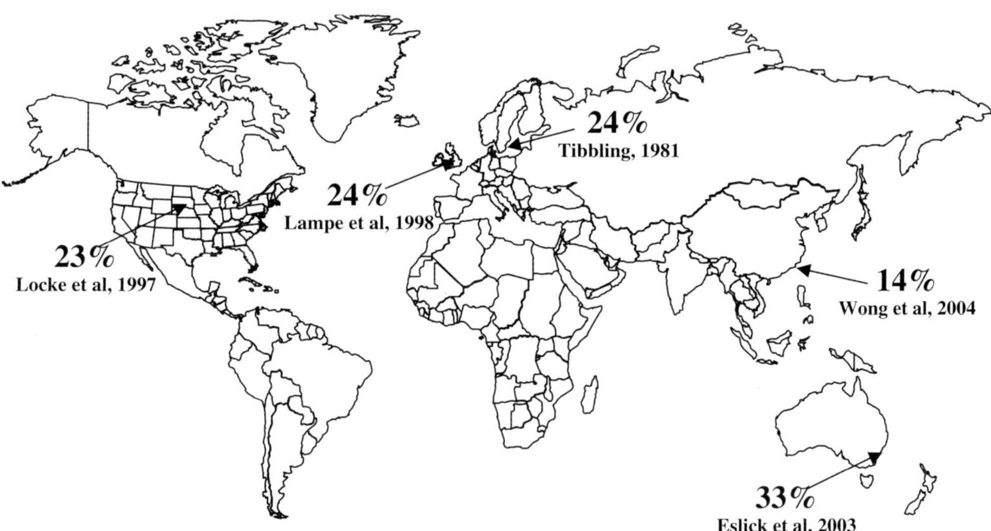

Fig 1–2. The community-based prevalence rates of noncardiac chest pain around the world.

be noted that a Swedish population-based longitudinal study of 321 individuals aged 53 to 87 years reported the prevalence of "chest pain" as 28%; however, noncardiac and cardiac cases were not differentiated. Therefore, this finding is not included as a population-based study assessing noncardiac chest pain.[13]

The first population-based study to determine the prevalence of noncardiac chest pain came from Sweden a quarter of a century ago.[11] It consisted of a survey which was cross-sectional in design conducted on a population of 3,000 individuals aged 25 to 55 years old to determine the prevalence of esophageal dysfunction (a proxy for noncardiac chest pain). The study reported that the prevalence of esophageal dysfunction in this community was 24% based on esophageal investigations (esophageal manometry and acid perfusion testing). Moreover, this study used a nonvalidated questionnaire with no mention about the contents of the questionnaire and no reference source provided.

It was more than a decade before the next population study appeared; it was from Olmsted County, Minnesota in the United States, with a focus on the clinical variety of gastroesophageal reflux disease.[9] This study consisted of 1,511 individuals who reported an overall prevalence of noncardiac chest pain of 23%; noncardiac chest pain was defined as "those who reported chest pain but did not have a history of cardiac disease."

The following year Lampe and colleagues from the United Kingdom published a population-based study of 7,735 randomly selected males aged 40 to 59 years, the prevalence of "other chest pain" was reported to be 24%[9]; the term "other chest pain' was based on examination by a nurse, exclusion of previous cardiac disease, and completion of the Rose Angina Questionnaire.[14]

More recent community-based studies from Australasia have provided a broad spectrum of prevalence rates for noncardiac chest pain compared to those previously undertaken around the world. However, both studies used the same definition for noncardiac chest pain over the same period (previous 12 months). An Australian study conducted in Sydney was specifically designed to assess the epidemiology of noncardiac chest pain in the general population.[8] It consisted of a sample of 1,000 individuals who were randomly selected from the electoral rolls and mailed the validated Chest Pain Questionnaire (CPQ), which had been purposely designed to examine the epidemiology of noncardiac chest pain.[15] The instrument measured chest pain symptoms, risk factors, psychological disorders, quality of life, and demographics. Noncardiac chest pain was defined as chest pain that was not angina (according to the Rose questionnaire criteria): (retrosternal pain precipitated by exertion and relieved by rest) that had not been diagnosed as due to ischemic heart disease by a physician. The study obtained an excellent response rate of 73% ($n =$ 672; mean age 46 years; 52% female). The study highlighted the heterogeneous nature of noncardiac chest pain (Fig 1–3). The authors reported that 33% ($n = 219$) of the subjects were classified as having noncardiac chest pain. Chest pain, however, was reported by 39% of the population; 7% reported a history of myocardial infarction, and 8% angina (based on the Rose Angina Questionnaire). The study also reported age and gender prevalence rates of noncardiac chest pain, which revealed that noncardiac chest pain decreases with increasing age. Females

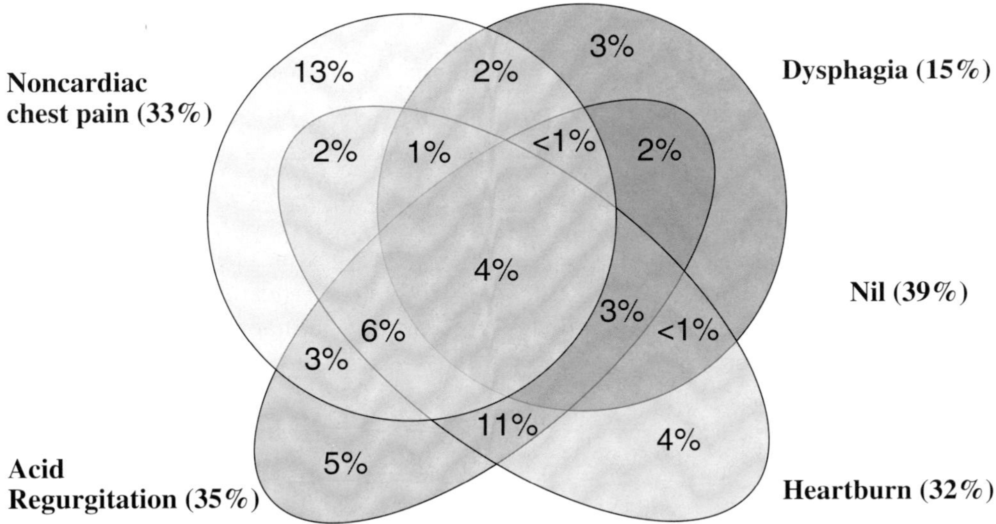

Note: numbers in parentheses are greater than and total more than 100% due to overlap.

Fig 1–3. Overlap among gastrointestinal symptoms and noncardiac chest pain. (Numbers in parentheses are greater than and total more than 100% due to overlap.)

aged between 50 to 59 years showed a statistically significant ($p = 0.04$) increase in noncardiac chest pain (Fig 1–4).

Wong and colleagues in Hong Kong conducted a community-based telephone survey of 2,209 Chinese households.[12] They used validated questionnaires, which included the Rose Angina Questionnaire, Gastroesophageal Reflux Questionnaire (GERQ), and the Hospital Anxiety and Depression Scale. Noncardiac chest pain was defined as nonexertional chest pain according to the Rose Angina Questionnaire and had not been diagnosed as ischemic heart disease by a physician. The prevalence of noncardiac chest pain was 13.9% ($n = 307$), and all chest pain was 20.6% ($n = 454$).

There are distinct differences among all these community-based studies, including how noncardiac chest pain was defined, sample size, sampling frame, questionnaires used, and ethnic and geo-graphic disparities. Conversely, there were also some important and consistent findings among these population-based studies. These include high prevalence rates of noncardiac chest pain (mean prevalence of these five studies: 23.6%) and very little if any difference in the prevalence of noncardiac chest pain between males and females. The most recent studies[8,12] used similar definitions for noncardiac chest pain, which gave widely different prevalence rates (14% vs 33%) of noncardiac chest pain. This disparity may be due to genetic/ethnic differences, sampling methods used, and the methods/instruments used (questionnaire vs telephone interview).

What does this mean in terms of the burden that noncardiac chest pain places on not just a community but an entire country? To show how this affects an entire population we calculate the population attributable risk (PAR). For example,

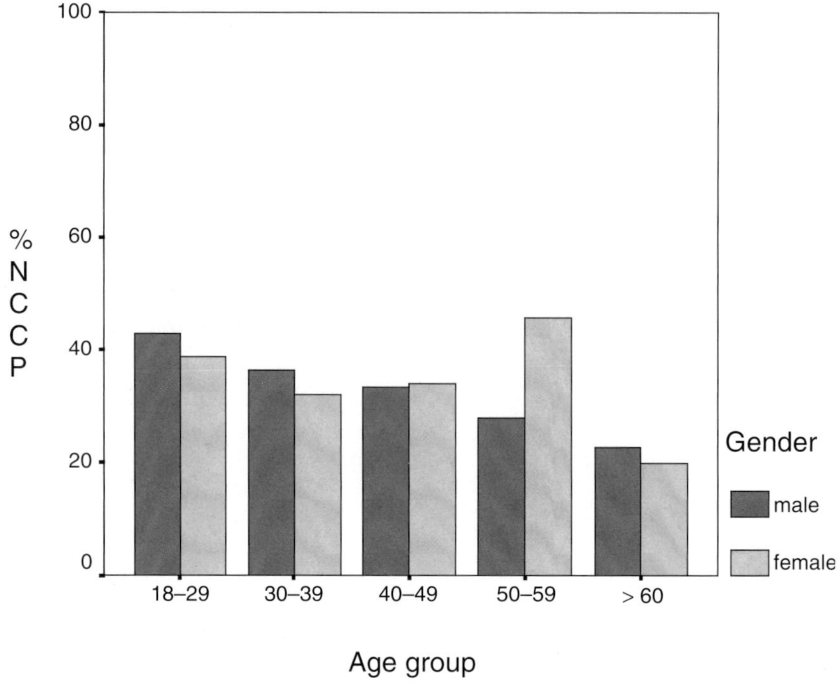

Fig 1–4. Population prevalence rates of noncardiac chest pain by age and gender (adapted from Eslick, Jones, & Talley[8]).

in the United States which has a current population of just over 300 million people, if we use a conservative prevalence estimate for noncardiac chest pain of 23%, this equates to approximately 69 million individuals who have noncardiac chest pain. This is an enormous number of individuals who are affected by an extremely debilitating condition, which has mammoth public health implications especially because a significant proportion of noncardiac chest pain is treatable.

Hospital-Based Studies

The majority of hospital-based studies assessing noncardiac chest pain have focused on determining the prevalence among patients who present to emer-gency departments or outpatient clinics with acute chest pain.[16] A few of these studies also aim to determine the cause of the patient's chest pain.[17,18]

Spalding and colleagues from the United Kingdom attempted to determine the cause of chest pain among 250 individuals who were admitted to hospital for chest pain.[18] Every patient was assessed as part of routine care and the discharge diagnosis provided from the medical records was the source of the diagnosis. Based on the initial classification of the 250 patients there were 142 (57%) with cardiac chest pain and 108 (43%) with "atypical chest pain." Patients with atypical chest pain were further classified into the following subgroups: musculoskeletal 25% ($n = 25$), cardiac 19% ($n = 21$), gastrointestinal 11% ($n = 12$), respiratory

9% ($n = 10$), and 37% ($n = 40$) were classified with an unknown cause for their chest pain. There were several limitations to this study, including, there was no specific definition for exactly what "atypical chest pain" was with the data collected from medical records and a follow-up questionnaire 1 year after admission. Moreover, the validity of the data may be questionable due to the potential for recall bias associated with using a questionnaire 12 months after admission as well as the lack of accuracy with regard to reporting made in the medical records.

One of the earliest studies reported was also one of the most comprehensive diagnostic assessments of chest pain patient's undertaken.[17] The study consisted of 204 nonacute myocardial infarction patients who underwent an extensive diagnostic examination to determine the cause of their acute chest pain. The diagnostic workup included an electrocardiogram ($n = 204$), exercise electrocardiogram ($n = 148$), myocardial scintigraphy ($n = 144$), Holter monitoring ($n = 136$), hyperventilation test ($n = 123$), echocardiography ($n = 146$), chest X-ray ($n = 204$), pulmonary scintigraphy ($n = 175$), esophagogastroduodenoscopy ($n = 133$), pH-monitoring in the esophagus ($n = 125$), Bernstein test ($n = 87$), physical examination of the chest wall ($n = 147$), bronchial histamine provocation test ($n = 147$), and ultrasonic examination of the abdomen ($n = 148$). The diagnostic workup of the patients revealed several clinical conditions including 42% ($n = 85$) with gastroesophageal diseases, 31% ($n = 64$) with ischemic heart disease, 28% ($n = 28$) with chest-wall syndromes, and the remainder of the patients being diagnosed with various conditions including pericarditis, pneumonia, pulmonary embolism, lung cancer, aortic aneurysm, aortic stenosis, and herpes zoster infection. Almost all the patients in the gastroesophageal disorders groups (89%, $n = 76/85$) had either an esophageal motility disorder (13%, $n = 26$) or gastroesophageal reflux disease (30%, $n = 62$). There was extensive overlap between cardiac and noncardiac diagnoses with 71% ($n = 144$) having a single diagnosis, 19% ($n = 39$) having two diagnoses, 2% ($n = 3$) having three diagnoses, and 8% ($n = 18$) with no diagnosis. The limitations of this study included the fact that older patients (>70 years) with severe heart failure were excluded, thus reducing the prevalence of those with ischemic heart disease. In addition, coronary angiography was not routinely performed in this study; a subset of patients ($n = 56$) received an incomplete diagnostic workup and therefore other possible diagnoses may have been missed; and no attempt was made to specify which diagnosis was important in terms of the chest pain.

Recently, a group from Japan conducted the first prevalence study of noncardiac chest pain among patients ($n = 952$) with recurrent chest-pain symptoms.[19] Four medical centers were involved in the recruitment of recurrent chest pain patients (the definition of recurrent chest pain was not mentioned in the article) undergoing coronary angiography investigation with the retrospective collection of both clinical and laboratory data from the medical records. Based on the coronary angiogram, patients were classified as having organic coronary heart disease and designated as having cardiac chest pain (CCP), whereas those without organic coronary disease were designated as having noncardiac chest pain. Sixty-six percent ($n = 633$) were found to have cardiac chest pain, whereas 34% ($n = 319$) were classified as having noncardiac chest pain. The findings of this study suggest that a substantial proportion of patients with recurrent chest pain in Japan have noncardiac chest pain.

Some studies focus on chest pain within certain subgroups of patients. Hendrix and colleagues in the United States conducted an analysis of the Hypertension Initiative database to determine the prevalence of chest pain syndromes among hypertensive patients.[20] The database contained 72,508 hypertensive patients and all disease classifications were made using the ICD-9. The authors reported that 11% of the hypertensive patients had a chest pain syndrome, with more than two-thirds (66%) diagnosed with only chest pain, 15% with angina, and 19% with an intermediate coronary syndrome (ICS). Moreover, it was reported that more females than males were diagnosed with chest pain only (86% vs 61%). It was concluded that chest pain is very common among hypertensive patients.

It can be observed from the above hospital-based studies that the potential causes of noncardiac chest pain are innumerable. There are many reasons for the differences found among these studies, including differences in ethnicity/genetics, country in which these studies are conducted, differences in the chest pain assessment protocol used, and the individual physicians' experience in treating and assessing acute chest pain.

General Practice Studies

Currently, there is only one General Practice study that has evaluated the natural history of patients diagnosed with chest pain of unspecified type or origin in primary care.[21] This was a population-based case-control study which assessed 13,740 patients with a first diagnosis of unspecified chest pain and 20,000 age- and sex-matched controls identified from the United Kingdom General Practice Research Database. The authors determined that the incidence rate of chest pain was 15.5 per 1,000 person-years and increased with age, particularly in men. The risk of a chest pain diagnosis was greatest in patients with prior diagnoses of coronary heart disease (OR: 7.1; 95% CI: 6.1-8.2) and gastroesophageal reflux disease (OR: 2.0; 95% CI: 1.7-2.3). In the year after diagnosis, chest pain patients were more likely than controls to be newly diagnosed with coronary heart disease (OR: 14.9; 95% CI: 12.7-17.4) and heart failure (OR: 4.7; 95% CI: 3.6-6.1). A new diagnosis of chest pain was associated with an increased risk of death in the following year (OR: 2.3; 95% CI: 1.9-2.8).

Qualitative Studies

A recent study of six combat veterans with chest pain who were admitted to a coronary care unit assessed the decision-making process related to seeking treatment for chest pain in a population of combat veterans with posttraumatic stress disorder and panic disorder.[22] Qualitative semistructured interviews were conducted to explore the veterans' prehospital experiences. The types of forces that affected combat veterans' decision-making process to seek medical treatment for chest pain symptoms were mainly "motivating" (feelings and appraisal of symptoms) rather than "restraining" (self-reliance, feelings, and appraisal of the symptoms, finances, mode of transportation, and past health care experiences). It was concluded that this group of individuals would not take action to seek treatment for chest pain until the "motivating forces" exceed the "restraining forces."

Pediatric Chest Pain

Chest pain is purported to be the second most common symptom associated with referral to a pediatric cardiologist and is rarely associated with fatal disease.[23-25] Chest pain among children and adolescents is analogous to chest pain among adults in that it has many varying causes (Fig 1-5).[26-38] Numerous studies have suggested that preponderance of chest pain among children and adolescents is noncardiac in origin.[39-42]

A prospective study of children (n = 50) aged 5 to 21 years referred to a cardiology clinic for assessment of chest pain were assessed for the causes of their chest pain.[40] All causes of chest pain were noncardiac in origin with the majority (76%) diagnosed with musculoskeletal pain, 12% having exercise-induced asthma, followed by 8% with gastrointestinal causes, and 4% having psychogenic causes. Lam and Tobias[41] conducted a 4-year follow-up study on 55 children and adolescents (27 females; 28 males) with a mean age of 14 years (range 6–20 years) who presented to a cardiology clinic for chest pain.[42] Causes of chest pain were varied with one-third idiopathic, 32% musculoskeletal, 15% gastroesophageal reflux disease, 8% supraventricular tachycardia, and the following representing 2% each: anxiety disorder, mitral valve prolapse, gastroesophageal reflux disease with anxiety, gastroesophageal reflux disease with musculoskeletal, and gastroesophageal reflux disease with hyperventilation. At 4-year follow-up, all the patients in this follow-up had noncardiac chest pain; just over half (51%) of the patients had no chest pain symptoms, whereas just under half (49%) had continued recurrent episodes of chest pain.

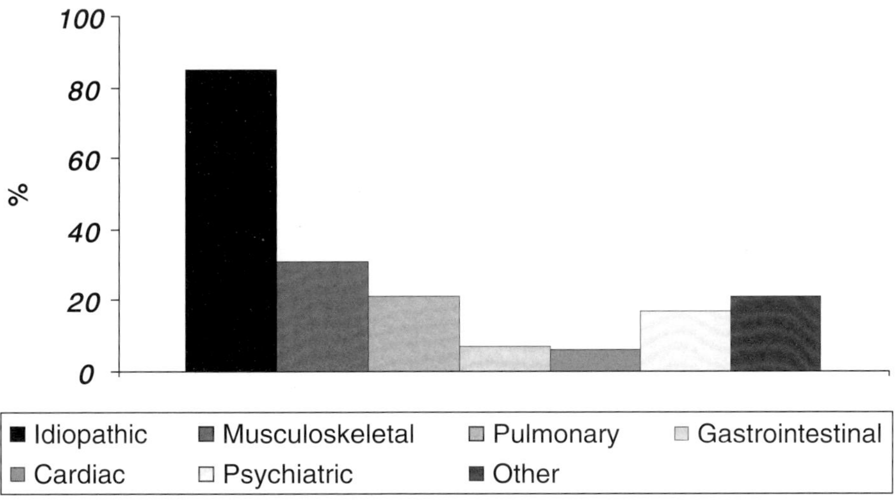

Fig 1–5. The potential causes of chest pain in children and adolescents.

Risk Factors

Currently, the risk factors associated with noncardiac chest pain remain poorly understood. Until recently there were no specific studies which had determined risk factors for noncardiac chest pain. Wise and colleagues from the Mayo Clinic in Rochester conducted a study to specifically examine risk factors among those with noncardiac chest pain in a community-based sample in the United States.[43] The validated Gastroesophageal Reflux Questionnaire (GERQ) was mailed out to 2,118 eligible individuals, with almost two-thirds (72%) returning the questionnaire. In addition, individuals who reported at least monthly or severe chest pain in response to a validated questionnaire were compared with healthy controls. Furthermore, medical records were reviewed and any individuals who had a relevant cardiac or organic disease were excluded. In total just over one-quarter (26%, $n = 389$) of individuals reported any chest pain and 12%, ($n = 186$) at least monthly or severe chest pain. Sixty-two individuals were excluded who had cardiac or organic conditions. Therefore, 124 individuals (9.1%, 95% CI: 7.6–10.8%) reported at least monthly or severe noncardiac chest pain, of which 65 (52.4%) had frequent reflux symptoms. There were a number of risk factors that were assessed in this sample including aspirin and NSAID use, smoking, coffee use, alcohol use, family history of reflux/heartburn, and body mass index (BMI). The authors reported several independent risk factors for noncardiac chest pain which included obesity (OR 3.0; 95% CI: 1.64–5.50), family history of reflux (OR 2.8; 95% CI: 1.73–4.32), previous cigarette use (OR 2.0; 95% CI: 1.27–3.18), aspirin use (OR 1.5; 95% CI: 1.00–2.31), and use of anti-arthritis medicines (OR 2.0; 95% CI: 1.27–3.16). Additional analysis found when comparing those with noncardiac chest pain and gastroesophageal reflux symptoms that those with noncardiac chest pain who did not have associated gastroesophageal reflux symptoms were less likely to have a family history of reflux, more likely to be younger, and less likely to be obese. Moreover, when comparing healthy controls with noncardiac chest pain sufferers, those with noncardiac chest pain without gastroesophageal reflux symptoms were younger (OR 0.97; 95% CI: 0.95–0.99), reported higher somatic symptom scores (OR 1.1; 95% CI: 1.08–1.73) and were more likely to be obese (OR 2.6; 95% CI: 1.15–5.93). Overall, this study found that risk factors for noncardiac chest pain are similar to risk factors for gastroesophageal reflux disease; this is because the individuals in the community who have substantial noncardiac chest pain also report frequent reflux symptoms. The study also reported that risk factors are different among those individuals who have noncardiac chest pain but no reflux symptoms.

It should be mentioned that other nonspecific studies have assessed potential risk factors among subgroups of noncardiac chest pain patients, for example, those with gastroesophageal reflux disease.[44,45] Additional probable risk factors for noncardiac chest pain might include certain foods and drinks (alcohol), smoking, menopause, stress, and pregnancy.[44-47] Due to the lack of dedicated studies specifically aimed to determine risk factors for noncardiac chest pain, additional studies are urgently required, especially those that concentrate on the modifiable lifestyle risk factors that can offer immediate relief to individuals who suffer with recurrent noncardiac chest pain.

Summary

Over the last decade the percentage of papers on noncardiac chest pain in the medical literature has produced a bimodal picture (Fig 1–6) with a peak in 2000 followed by a decline in the number of articles on noncardiac chest pain. Recently, this picture has changed once again with an increase in the number of articles on the topic since 2004, suggesting an increased interest in this important medical condition.

Currently, the epidemiology of noncardiac chest pain remains poorly understood, with an urgent need for quality studies that use a priori hypotheses, appropriate methodology, and acceptable definition(s) for noncardiac chest pain. There is a necessity for more population-based studies from different countries which should also determine potential risk factors for those with noncardiac chest pain. Based on the handful of community-based studies available, the prevalence of noncardiac chest pain is around 25%. The natural history of noncardiac chest pain in the community has not been sufficiently investigated. There are several hospital-based studies that have highlighted the fact that noncardiac chest pain is a heterogeneous condition; however, there is still great difficulty in differentiating noncardiac from cardiac chest pain and other fatal causes of chest pain in a proportion of patients who present with acute chest pain to emergency departments. There is also a lack of primary care-based studies in General Practice and among the pediatric population where both groups should receive prolonged follow-up and continued monitoring. Risk factors associated with noncardiac

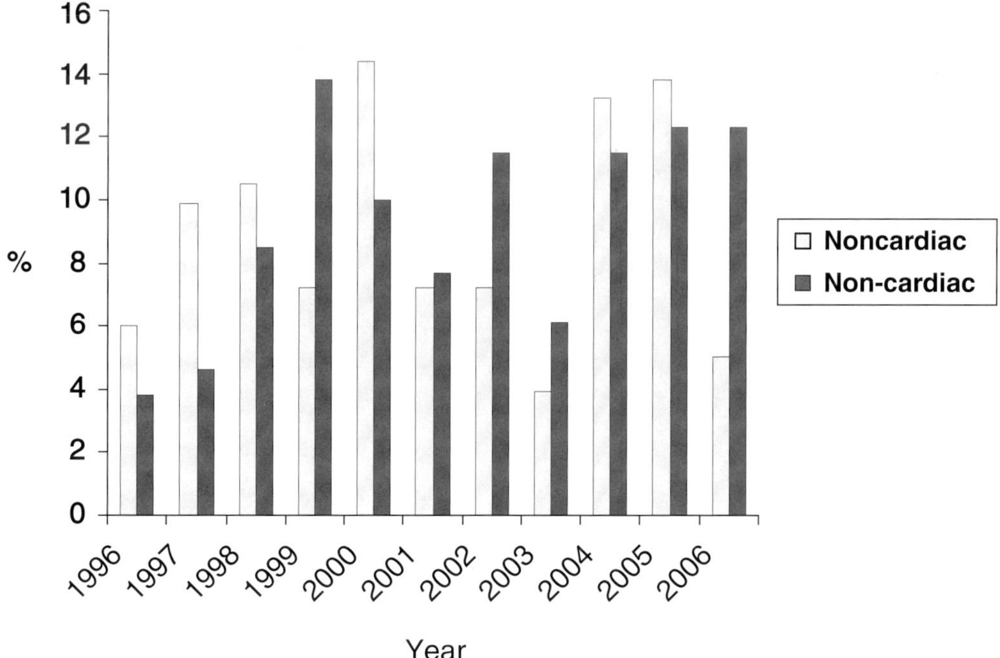

Fig 1–6. MEDLINE search of "noncardiac chest pain" and "non-cardiac chest pain" from 1996 to 2006.

chest pain require further elucidation both within the community and hospital-based subjects. Epidemiologic studies into noncardiac chest pain have made great progress over the last few years and one hopes future studies will provide much new data and information on this important medical condition.

References

1. Eslick GD. Chest pain: an historical perspective. *Int J Cardiol.* 2001;77:5–11.
2. Heberden W. Some account of a disorder of the breast. *Med Trans Roy Coll Phys Lond.* 1772;2:59–67.
3. Gilmiche JP, Clouse RE, Balint A, Cook IJ, Kahrilas PJ, Paterson WG, Smount AJMP. Functional esophageal disorders. *Gastroenterology.* 2006;130:1459–1465.
4. Boyce PM, Talley NJ, Burke C, Koloski NA. Epidemiology of the functional gastrointestinal disorders diagnosed according to Rome II criteria: an Australian population-based study. *Intern Med J.* 2006; 36:28–36.
5. Koloski NA, Talley NJ, Boyce PM. The impact of functional gastrointestinal disorders on quality of life. *Am J Gastroenterol.* 2000;95:67–71.
6. Koloski NA, Talley NJ, Boyce PM. Epidemiology and health care seeking in the functional GI disorders: a population-based study. *Am J Gastroenterol.* 2002; 97:2290–2299.
7. Kachintorn U. How do we define noncardiac chest pain? *J Gastroenterol Hepatol.* 2005;20(suppl):S2–S5.
8. Eslick GD, Jones MP, Talley NJ. Noncardiac chest pain: prevalence, risk factors, impact and consulting—a population-based study. *Aliment Pharmacol Ther.* 2003;17:1115–1124.
9. Lampe FC, Whincup PH, Wannamethee SG, Ebrahim S, Walker M, Shaper AG. Chest pain on questionnaire and prediction of major ischaemic heart disease events in men. *Eur Heart J.* 1998;19: 63–73.
10. Locke GR 3rd, Talley NJ, Fett SL, Zinsmeister AR, Melton JL. Prevalence and clinical spectrum of gastro-oesophageal reflux: a population-based study in Olmsted County, Minnesota. *Gastroenterology.* 1997;112:1448–1456.
11. Tibbling L. Oesophageal dysfunction and angina pectoris in a Swedish population selected at random. *Acta Medica Scandinavia.* 1981:644(suppl):71–74.
12. Wong WM, Lam KF, Cheng C, et al. Population based study of noncardiac chest pain in southern Chinese: prevalence, psychosocial factors and health care utilization. *World J Gastroenterol.* 2004;10: 707–712.
13. Brattberg G, Parker MG, Thorslund M. A longitudinal study of pain: reported pain from middle age to old age. *Clin J Pain.* 1997;13:144–149.
14. Rose G. The diagnosis of ischaemic heart pain and intermittent claudication in field surveys. *Bull World Health Organ.* 1962;27:645–658.
15. Eslick GD, Talley NJ. The development and validation of the Chest Pain Questionnaire (CPQ) for non-cardiac chest pain (NCCP). *Gastroenterology.* 2004;126(suppl 2): A-309.
16. Eslick GD, Coulshed DS, Talley NJ. Diagnosis and treatment of noncardiac chest pain. *Nat Clin Pract Gastroenterol Hepatol.* 2005;2:463–472.
17. Fruergaard P, Launbjerg J, Hesse B, et al. The diagnosis of patients admitted with acute chest pain but without myocardial infarction. *Eur Heart J.* 1996;17:1028–1034.
18. Spalding L, Reay E, Kelly C. Cause and outcome of atypical chest pain in patients admitted to hospital. *J Royal Soc Med.* 2003;96:122–125.
19. Imaoka T, Miyaoka Y, Nishi K, et al. Prevalence of noncardiac chest pain in Japanese patients with recurrent chest pain. *J Gastroenterol.* 2005;40:913–914.

20. Hendrix KH, Mayhan S, Lackland DT, Egan BM. Prevalence, treatment, and control of chest pain syndromes and associated risk factors in hypertensive patients. *Am J Hypertension*. 2005;18:1026-1032.

21. Ruigomez A, Rodriguez LAG, Wallander M-A, Johansson S, Jones R. Chest pain in general practice: incidence, comorbidity and mortality. *Fam Pract*. 2006;23: 167-174.

22. Alcaras NM, Roper JM. Chest pain among combat veterans: conceptual framework. *Military Med*. 2006;171:478-483.

23. Balfour IC, Syamasudar Rao P. Chest pain in children. *Ind J Pediatr*. 1998;65:21-26.

24. Brenner JI, Ringel RE, Berman MA. Cardiologic perspectives of chest pain in childhood: a referral problem? To whom? *Pediatr Clin North Am*. 1984;31: 1241-1258.

25. Kocis KC. Chest pain in pediatrics. *Pediatr Clin North Am*. 1999;46:189-203.

26. Coleman W. Recurrent chest pain in children. *Pediatr Clin North Am*. 1984;31(5) 1007-1026.

27. Driscoll DJ, Glicklich LB, Gallen WJ. Chest pain in children: a prospective study. *Pediatrics*. 1976;57:648-651.

28. Fyfe MD. Chest pain in pediatric patients presenting to a cardiac clinic. *Clin Pediatrics*. 1984;23:321-340.

29. Gutgesell HP, Barst RJ, Humes RA, et al. Common cardiovascular problems in the young: Part I. Murmurs, chest pain, syncope and irregular rhythms. *Am Fam Phys*. 1997;567:1825-1830.

30. Leung AK, Robson WL, Cho H. Chest pain in children. *Can Fam Phys*. 1996; 42:1163-1164.

31. Milov DE, Kantor RJ. Chest pain in teenagers. *Postgraduate Med*. 1990;885: 145-154.

32. Pantell RH, Goodman BW. Adolescent chest pain: a prospective study. *Pediatrics*. 1983;716:881-887.

33. Perry RF, Garlisi AP, Allison EJ, et al. Acute myocardial infarction in a 16-year-old boy with no predisposing risk factors. *Pediatr Emerg Care*. 1997;136: 413-416.

34. Selbst S. Chest pain in children. *Pediatrics*. 1985;756:1068-1070.

35. Selbst SM. Evaluation of chest pain in children. *Pediatr Rev*. 1986;82:56-62.

36. Selbst SM, Ruddy RM, Clark BJ. Pediatric chest pain: a prospective study. *Pediatrics*. 1988;823:319-323.

37. Selbst SM, Ruddy RM, Clark BJ. Chest pain in children. *Clin Pediatrics*. 1990; 297:374-377.

38. Swenson JM, Fischer DR, Miller SA, et al. Are chest pain radiographs and electocardiograms still valuable in evaluating new pediatric patients with heart murmurs or chest pain? *Pediatrics*. 1997; 991:1-3.

39. Talner NS, Carboni MP. Chest pain in the adolescent and young adult. *Cardiol Rev*. 2000;8:49-56.

40. Evangelista JA, Parsons M, Renneberg AK. Chest pain in children: diagnosis through history and physical examination. *J Pediatr Health Care*. 2000;14:3-8.

41. Lam JC, Tobias JD. Follow-up survey of children and adolescents with chest pain. *Southern Med J*. 2001;94:921-924.

42. Sabri MR, Ghavanimi AA, Haghighat M, Imanieh MH. Chest pain in children and adolescents: epigastric tenderness as a guide to reduce unnecessary work-up. *Pediatr Cardiol*. 2003;24:3-5.

43. Wise JL, Locke GR. Zinsmeister AR, Talley NJ. Risk factors for non-cardiac chest pain in the community. *Aliment Pharmacol Ther*. 2005;22:1023-1031.

44. Bolin TD, Korman MG, Hansky J, Stanton R. Heartburn: community perceptions. *J Gastroenterol Hepatol*. 1999;15:35-39.

45. Oliveria SA, Christos PJ, Talley NJ, Dannenberg AJ. Heartburn risk factors, knowledge, and prevention strategies. *Arch Intern Med*. 1999;159:1592-1598.

46. Asplund R, Aberg HE. Nightmares, cardiac symptoms and the menopause. *Climacteric*. 2003;6:314-320.

47. Rosano GMC, Collins P, Kaski JC, Lindsay DC, Sarrel PM, Poole-Wilson PA. Syndrome X in women is associated with oestrogen deficiency. *Eur Heart J*. 1995; 16:610-614.

CHAPTER 2

Evaluation of Chest Pain

A Cardiology Perspective for the Gastroenterologist

Paul E. Fenster
Vincent L. Sorrell

A cardiologist is often the first physician to see a patient with chest pain, whether the origin is cardiac or noncardiac. As many as 55% of patients who report to an emergency room with chest pain or other symptoms suggestive of acute cardiac ischemia have noncardiac problems,[1] and approximately 30% of patients evaluated for chest pain by coronary angiography each year show no evidence of coronary artery disease.[2]

The cardiologist's first priority is to exclude any acute life-threatening cardiovascular condition. Then, the patient should be evaluated for chronic ischemic heart disease or pericardial disease. Once these have been ruled out as possible causes of chest pain, a diagnosis of noncardiac chest pain (NCCP) is made, and the patient is treated for NCCP or referred to a gastroenterologist or other specialist for follow-up. An understanding of NCCP from the cardiology and gastroenterology perspectives is necessary for effective management of this disorder. Many of these patients repeatedly return to the emergency department if the gastrointestinal disorder is not adequately treated or if they do not understand that their symptoms are not signs of an impending heart attack.[3] On the other hand, a missed diagnosis of a cardiac event can have serious consequences. The overlap in symptoms for cardiovascular disease and NCCP can make accurate diagnosis difficult, and highlights the need for collaboration on the part of both these specialties.

The Cardiac Esophageal Connection and Cardioesophageal Reflexes

Cardioesophageal reflexes are responsible for a number of clinically important phenomena. There is strong evidence that events that occur in the esophagus can alter cardiac function, particularly the coronary circulation.[4] There is also evidence that coronary events can alter esophageal function.[5]

Stimulation of the esophagus by acid, distention, or hot or cold liquids can produce changes in the coronary vasculature and in cardiac rhythm. The change in rhythm is most commonly vagally mediated, and the bradycardia that results can be sinus bradycardia or atrioventricular nodal block of varying degrees. Acid infusion into the esophagus can decrease coronary blood flow in normal coronary arteries. This is not due to a vagal mechanism. The cause is uncertain. Ischemic pain that is triggered by digestive factors has been termed "linked angina."

Linked angina was explored by Chauhan et al[4] in 35 patients with syndrome X and in 24 patients who had received a heart transplant. The transplanted heart is denervated. Patients with syndrome X have typical angina and objective evidence of cardiac ischemia but have angiographically normal epicardial coronary arteries. The presumed explanation for their pain is that there is an abnormality in the function of the small coronary arteries, the microvasculature, despite normal large coronary arteries. An array of abnormalities, including nitric oxide deficiency, endothelial cell dysfunction, angiotensin II type I receptor up-regulation, and increased sympathetic tone, have been found in these patients.

In the Chauhan study, all the syndrome X patients had a history of typical angina, a positive exercise echo, and normal coronary arteries on angiography. In these patients, esophageal infusion of hydrochloric acid significantly reduced coronary blood flow as measured by an intracoronary Doppler flow catheter. In contrast, acid infusion had no effect on coronary blood flow in the heart transplant group.[4] Twenty (57%) of the 35 syndrome X patients experienced ischemic pain provoked by the infusion of acid, but there were no changes in heart rate or blood pressure, eliminating a hemodynamic response as the cause. In the 15 patients who did not experience pain, no change was noted in coronary blood flow. In the 20 patients with pain, a significant decrease in flow was observed—from 85 mL per minute to 36 mL per minute.[4] No change was seen in the angiographically measured size of the left anterior descending coronary artery, so coronary artery spasm was not involved.[4] Thus, microvascular dysfunction was implicated as the cause of reduced blood flow and chest pain, in response to acid infusion, in 57% of these patients with syndrome X. Furthermore, on the basis of its absence in patients who had transplanted, denervated hearts, linked angina would seem to be a neurally mediated cardioesophageal reflex mechanism that occurs only in susceptible patients.[4]

Cardiac events may have an effect on esophageal function. During coronary angiography and angioplasty, changes in esophageal function often occur. In 30 stable patients undergoing elective cardiac catheterization to determine the cause of chest pain, of whom four required angioplasty, esophageal manometry and esophageal pH were monitored throughout the cardiac procedure.[5] Afterward, esophageal provocation with ice water, hydrochloric acid, and balloon inflation were performed along with observation of cardiac rate and rhythm. Five of 13 patients with normal coronary arteries developed esophageal spasm during coronary angiography, as did 5 of 17 patients with abnormal coronary arteries.[5] No changes in esophageal pH occurred during cardiac catheterization, indicating that acid reflux was not a cause of pain, and neither cardiac rate nor rhythm changed during esophageal manipulation.[5]

Although chest pain is not usually a consequence of angiography, it may occur in patients undergoing angioplasty, presumably due to the transient ischemia induced by the procedure itself. These findings imply that the pain that occurs during coronary artery procedures may be, in part, the result of esophageal spasm.

Cardiac Assessments

The pain caused by a cardiac event may occur anywhere from the patient's nose to the navel. When a patient presents with chest pain, the first priority is to assess the probability of a life-threatening situation. These conditions include acute myocardial infarction, unstable angina, aortic dissection, pulmonary thromboembolism, and pericardial tamponade.

These conditions usually can be diagnosed quickly by a carefully obtained history, thorough physical examination, electrocardiogram, chest radiograph, and blood tests, including cardiac markers (troponin) or cardiac enzymes. The subsequent assessment may point to the need for an echocardiogram, nuclear scan, chest computed tomography or magnetic resonance imaging, or cardiac catheterization. Life-threatening conditions usually can be detected, and treatment initiated, within hours of the patient's presentation.

Even if an acute cardiac syndrome has been deemed unlikely, it is usually necessary to determine if pain is cardiac in origin. Chronic, stable cardiac conditions carry an increased risk of myocardial infarction over the long term because cardiovascular diseases are progressive. The presence of myocardial ischemia can be confirmed through provocative testing. However, the cause of the patient's chest pain may not be related to the ischemia as ischemia and chest pain can coexist without a causal relationship. Certainly, there is no substitute for a carefully obtained history to help in these circumstances.

The description of chest pain obtained during a careful history is categorized as typical angina (80–90% likelihood of obstructive coronary artery disease), atypical angina (40–80% likelihood), or as noncardiac (20–70% likelihood). Typical angina is characterized by the following three characteristics: (1) retrosternal chest discomfort experienced as pressure or heaviness; (2) duration of 5 to 15 minutes; and (3) induced by stress or exertion, a large meal, or exposure to cold and relieved by rest or nitroglycerin. Atypical angina is diagnosed when two of these are present, and noncardiac pain is likely if none, or only one, of these cardinal features exist. Therefore, a patient who describes the spontaneous onset of "an elephant sitting on my chest" for 1 minute, with left arm involvement, diaphoresis, and nausea actually has noncardiac chest pain.

Although some patients have a high probability of cardiac origin for their chest pain and others have a low probability, a great number of patients fall into the intermediate range. Bayesian logic dictates that these intermediate probability patients will benefit the most from provocative testing with exercise, or with pharmacologic agents when exercise is not possible. The severity and extent of ischemia, the left ventricular function, the appearance of the coronary arteries, and the functional capacity are determined using modern imaging devices and permit an accurate estimate of a patient's prognosis. Treadmill electrocardiographic (ECG) stress testing, with or without myocardial perfusion nuclear SPECT and echocardiographic (echo) imaging, is the mainstay of provocative ischemic testing. When patients cannot perform adequate exercise to "stress the heart" (exercise to a level that would create a myocardial oxygen supply/demand mismatch in the presence of impaired coronary flow), then pharmacologic testing is required. In these circumstances, ECG monitoring alone is not adequate to identify ischemia and testing is combined with either SPECT or echo (Figs 2–1 and

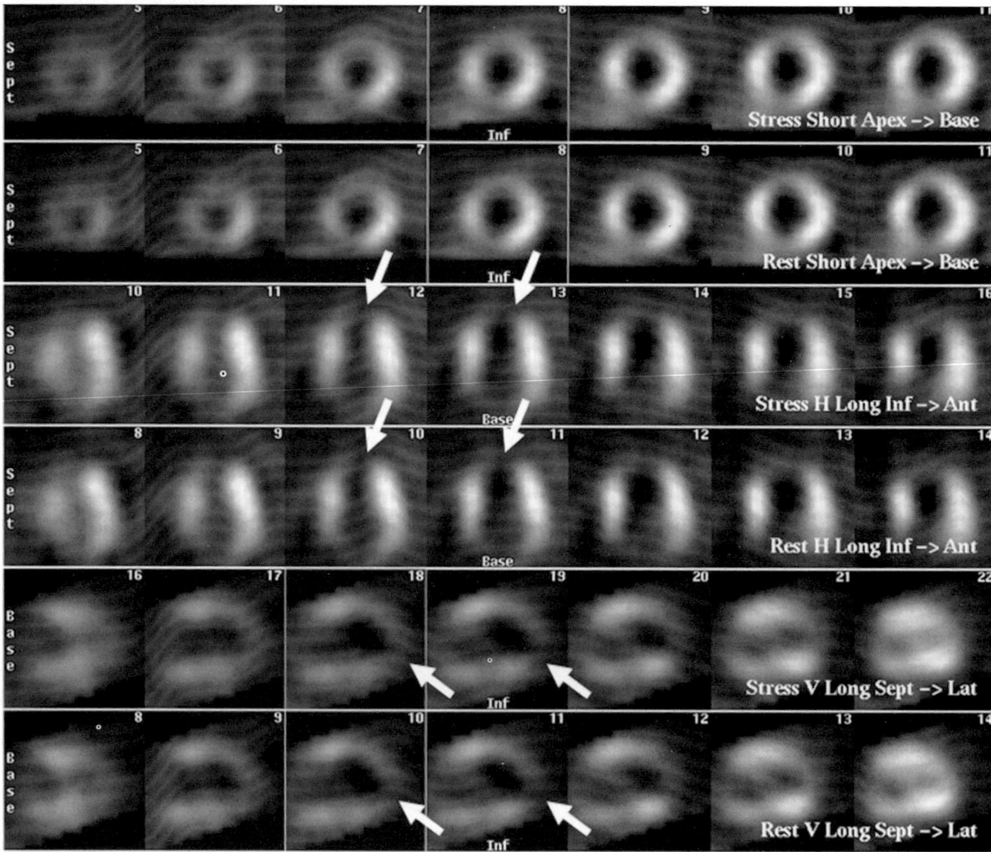

Fig 2–1. Nuclear SPECT myocardial perfusion imaging exam in a patient with chest pain. Each pair of rows represents the stress and rest myocardial perfusion images. Note radiotracer distribution is normal (*white*) in all regions except the left ventricular apex (*arrows*). As this is in both the rest and stress data sets, it most likely represents a previous apical infarction.

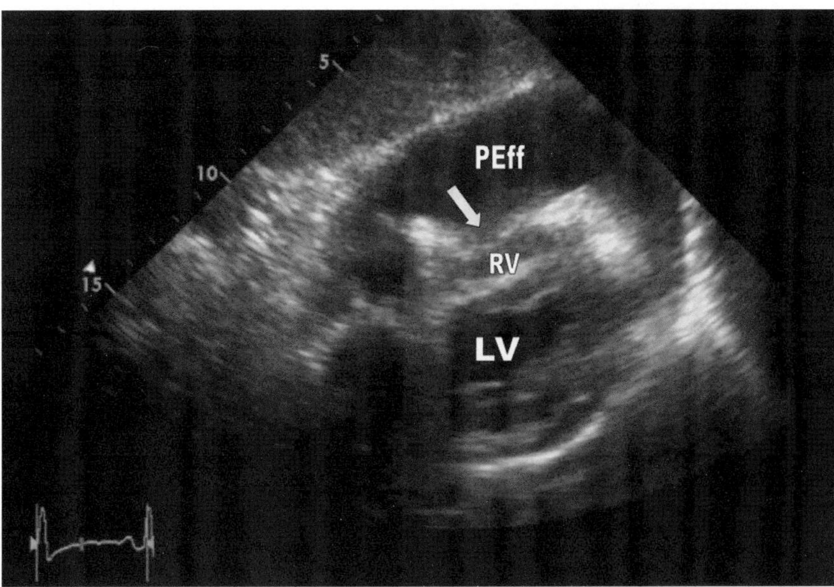

Fig 2–2. Transthoracic two-dimensional echocardiogram in a patient with chest pain, oriented from a subcostal imaging window (liver on top of image). A large black space is noted (PEff = pericardial effusion) and this compressed the RV cavity (*arrow*) consistent with cardiac tamponade. RV = right ventricle; LV = left ventricle.

2-2). The use of pharmacologic testing is now required in more than 50% of patients who are being evaluated for myocardial ischemia.

Although a normal test result never entirely excludes coronary artery disease as the etiology of a chest pain syndrome, it does indicate an excellent prognosis. A normal or mildly abnormal test result has an overwhelmingly good prognosis, regardless of the underlying coronary anatomy. Additionally, a markedly abnormal test result indicates a poor prognosis, even when the coronary anatomy is normal or mildly stenotic by angiography.

A new crop of modern tests has been developed to specifically assist in the evaluation of the patient with a suspected cardiac origin of chest pain. These include cardiac CT (CCT) and MRI (CMR) (Figs 2-3 and 2-4). Although an exhaustive description of these sophisticated imaging tools is beyond the scope of this chapter, a brief review is indicated as these imaging modalities offer novel perspectives on cardiac pathology and will continue to account for a greater percentage of testing. CMR has quickly become the new reference standard for LV (and RV) function. CCT is the noninvasive approach for diagnostic coronary angiography and is replacing the traditional invasive coronary angio-gram (which remains the reference standard). Recently, the appropriateness criteria guidelines were established to assist referring physicians as to the published indications for these tools.[6,7]

In many ways, CCT is similar to nuclear SPECT imaging. Both tools expose the

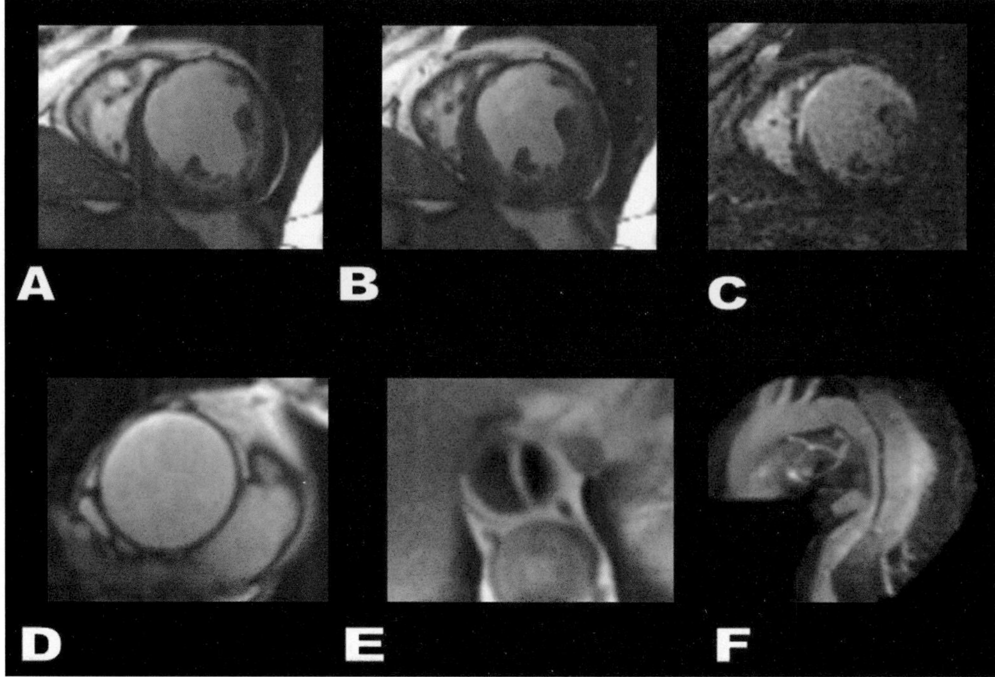

Fig 2–3. Cardiac MRI exam in a patient with chest pain. Short-axis image of the LV in diastole (*A*) and systole (*B*) shows a large LV cavity, thin anteroseptal wall which does not move in systole. The viability sequence confirms that the anteroseptal wall is infarcted (*C*; white = scarring). The ascending aorta (white blood sequence) is mildly dilated (*D*). The descending aorta (black blood sequence) confirms that a dissection is present (*E*). The thin white line bisecting the aorta is the dissected intima. With contrast enhancement, 3D angiographic images are obtained and confirm a large Type II dissection (*F*).

patient to radiation, both tools obtain the "raw" data quickly, but require extensive off-line processing prior to final interpretation, and both have an excellent negative predictive capability and relatively high false-positive rate. Nuclear SPECT focuses on the myocardial perfusion (blood flow) and CCT focuses on the coronary anatomy (calcium and stenosis). Also, both tools are subject to artifacts from irregular rhythms and incorrect processing of the source data.

Similarly, CMR is more closely linked with stress echocardiography. Both of these tools are nonradiating, essentially real-time exams without extensive post-processing required, and more resistant to rhythm disturbances. Both have excellent capabilities of evaluating the ventricular sizes and function, and valve physiology, as well as a high specificity for myocardial ischemia and scarring. Both of these imaging tools are extremely comprehensive, which is why there are ~25 million echo exams performed annually.[8] CMR is frequently combined with dobutamine to assess wall motion changes or with a vasodilator to assess blood flow changes making this tool the most versatile of all imaging modalities.

It is critical to remember that the patient's history should remain the principal

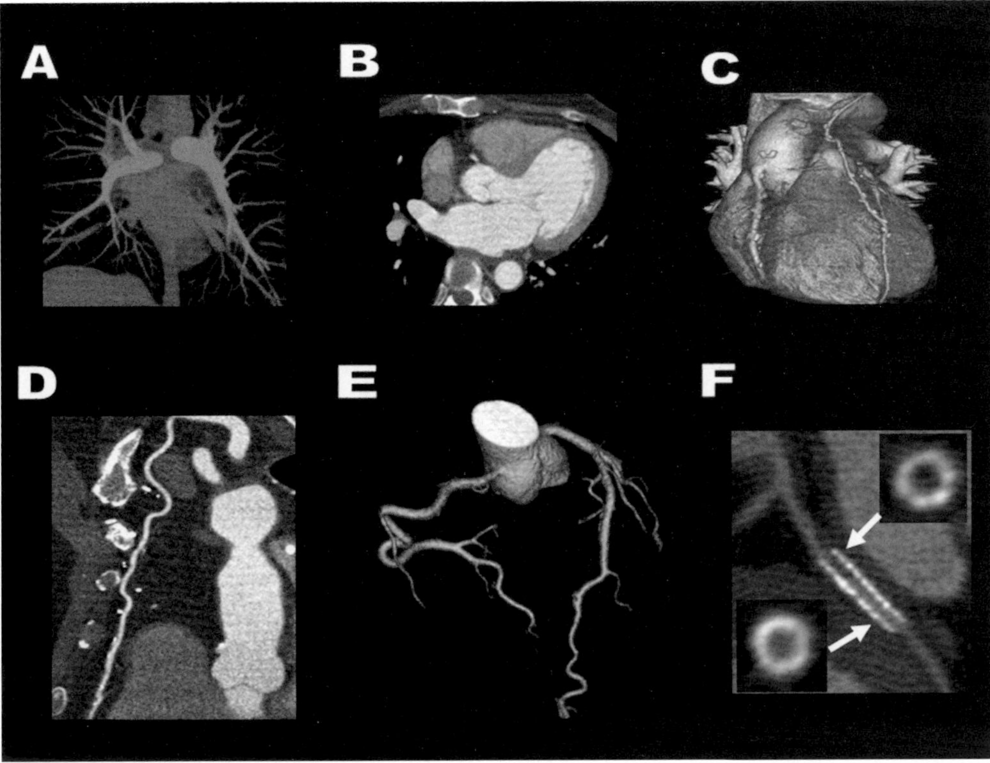

Fig 2–4. Multislice cardiac CT scan in a patient with chest pain. 3D pulmonary angiogram without evidence for a pulmonary emboli (*A*). Gated multiphasic reconstruction images provide an accurate assessment of LV function and wall motion (*B*). 3D volume rendered image shows the details of the cardiac structures and the coronary bypass grafts (*C*). Multiplanar reconstructed images allow the bypassed internal mammary artery to be carefully evaluated from its origin to the coronary anastomosis (*D*). Additional image processing allows one to display only the native coronary arteries (*E*). Recent data suggests that CT imaging may even allow the assessment of intracoronary stent patency and restenosis as shown in panel *F*. Restenosis is suggested by the lack of contrast (*dark center*) in the proximal stent (*upper right panel*) versus the patent stent (brighter center) in the distal stent (*lower left panel*). Images courtesy of Dr. Tamar Gaspar, Lady Davis Carmel Medical Center, Haifa, Israel.

determinant of how to proceed after any test result. A patient with an intermediate to high pretest likelihood of having coronary artery disease and a normal test result likely has coronary artery disease and requires aggressive risk factor modification and close follow-up. If symptoms continue, the patient should undergo invasive coronary angiography, despite the normal test result. Furthermore, the patient with a low to intermediate pretest likelihood of having coronary artery disease, a normal or mild-moderately abnormal stress test result, and with continued chest pain may benefit from a CCT.

Given the proliferation of imaging options for evaluating the etiology of chest pain, it is important to know what expertise is locally available. An expertly performed stress echocardiogram will always be a more valuable test than a low-quality nuclear test, and vice versa. If this is not known, or if there are experts in all imaging modalities available, then a working algorithm for choosing the most appropriate test will increase the yield of diagnostic tests. One such algorithm is provided in Figure 2–5.

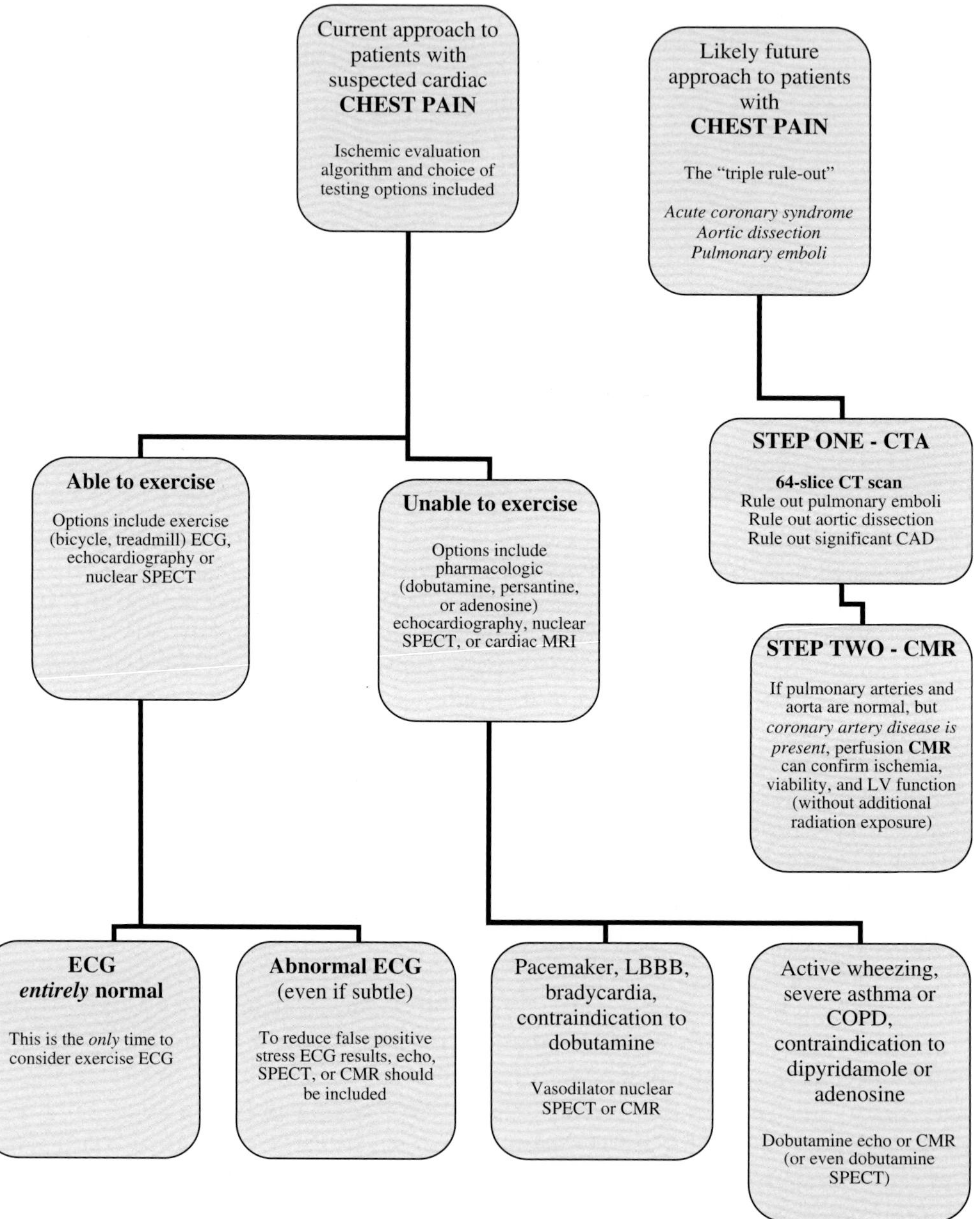

Fig 2–5. Working Algorithm for Selecting Appropriate Diagnostic Tests for Evaluation of Chest Pain.

Treatment of NCCP

If the pain is determined to be noncardiac in nature, most cardiologists refer the patient to a gastroenterologist or primary care physician for further evaluation. In many cases, the cardiologist may prescribe an H_2-receptor antagonist or a proton-pump inhibitor (PPI) because there is a common belief that most NCCP is acid reflux related.

Summary

Evidence indicates that there is a clinically significant cardioesophageal connection in patients who experience esophageal or ischemic problems. Cardiologists and gastroenterologists often find the coexistence of symptoms and functional abnormalities, but determining causation is much more difficult. There is a need for better understanding of the phenomenon of cardiac and NCCP, among cardiologists and gastroenterologists.

In evaluating chest pain, the cardiologist assesses the probability that the condition is acute and life threatening; serious and chronic; or noncardiac in nature. If it seems to be cardiac chest pain, appropriate therapy is initiated. In patients in whom there is a strong suspicion of NCCP, a PPI is often prescribed, or the patient is referred to a gastroenterologist or a primary care physician for further evaluation.

References

1. Pope JH, Aufderheide TP, Ruthazer R, et al. Missed diagnoses of acute cardiac ischemia in the emergency department. *N Engl J Med.* 2000:342:1163–1170.
2. Katz PO, Castell DO. Approach to the patient with unexplained chest pain. *Am J Gastroenterol.* 2000;95(suppl 8):S4–S8.
3. Richter JE, Bradley LA, Castell DO. Esophageal chest pain: current controversies in pathogenesis, diagnosis, and therapy. *Ann Intern Med.* 1989;110: 66–78.
4. Chauhan A, Petch MC, Schofield PM. Cardio-esophageal reflex in humans as a mechanism for "linked angina." *Eur Heart J.* 1996;17:407–413.
5. Makk JL, Leesar M, Joseph A, Prince CP, Wright RA. Cardioesophageal reflexes: an invasive human study. *Dig Dis Sci.* 2000;45:2451–2454.
6. Hendel RC, Patel MR, Kramer CM, et al. for the ACCF/ACR/SCCT/SCMR/ASNC/ NASCI/SCAI/SIR societies. 2006 appropriateness criteria for cardiac computed tomography and cardiac magnetic resonance imaging. *J Am Coll Cardiol.* 2006; 48(7):1475–1497.
7. Brindis RG, Douglas PS, Hendel RC, et al. for the ACCF/ASNC societies. 2005 appropriateness criteria for single-photon emission computed tomography myocardial perfusion imaging (SPECT MPI). *J Am Coll Cardiol.* 2005;46(8):1587–1605. Erratum in: *J Am Coll Cardiol.* 2005; 46(11):2148–2150.
8. Arlington Medical Resources, Inc. *The Echocardiography Market Guide* (USA). July–December 2005.

CHAPTER 3

Pathophysiology of Noncardiac Chest Pain

Ronnie Fass
Jae Geun Hyun
Justin L. Sewell

Introduction

The pathophysiology of NCCP remains to be fully elucidated. Identified underlying mechanisms are diverse and often overlap. Gastroesophageal reflux disease (GERD) is by far the most common cause of NCCP. Other etiologic factors that have been proposed include esophageal motility disorders, abnormal mechanophysical properties of the esophagus, sustained longitudinal muscle contractions, visceral hypersensitivity, altered central processing of intraesophageal stimuli, altered autonomic activity, and psychological comorbidity (Table 3-1). Whereas some of the proposed underlying mechanisms have been well substantiated, others suffer from paucity of data demonstrating clear causality.

Table 3–1. The Different Proposed Underlying Mechanisms of Noncardiac Chest Pain

- Gastroesophageal reflux
- Esophageal dysmotility
- Abnormal mechanophysical properties
  - Hyperactive
  - ↓ Reduced compliance
- Sustained longitudinal muscle contractions
- Visceral hypersensitivity
- Altered central processing of visceral stimuli
- Altered autonomic activity
- Psychological abnormalities
  - Panic attack
  - Anxiety
  - Depression

GERD

GERD has been reported to be the most common underlying mechanism for NCCP. Between 25 to 60% of patients with noncardiac chest pain have demonstrated abnormal 24-hour esophageal pH monitoring and/or positive upper endoscopy findings. Typical GERD symptoms, heartburn and acid regurgitation, were found to be significantly and independently associated with the presence of NCCP. Locke et al[1] demonstrated that NCCP was reported more often by patients experiencing frequent heartburn symptoms (at least once a week) as compared to those with infrequent heartburn symptoms (less than once a week) and individuals reporting no GERD symptoms. Eslick et al[2] performed a population-based study to determine the prevalence of NCCP. The authors found that among subjects with NCCP, 53% experienced heartburn, and 58% acid regurgitation.

The findings of esophageal erosions on upper endoscopy in patients with GERD-related NCCP have been reported to range between 10 and 70%.[3,4] The different patient populations evaluated can explain the wide range of the results.

Abnormal ambulatory 24-hour esophageal pH monitoring is demonstrated in approximately 50% of patients with NCCP. Fass et al[5] reported that 41.1% of 37 patients with NCCP had abnormal pH tests. Beedassy et al[6] evaluated 104 patients with NCCP and reported that 48% had an abnormal pH test. Of the total number of patients in the study, 52 reported chest pain during the pH study, but only 23 (44%) had an abnormal pH test. In this group of NCCP patients, only 21% reported chest pain that coincided with an abnormal pH test.

A positive (>50%) symptom index (percentage of symptoms associated acid reflux events) in NCCP patients with normal pH test has been considered indicative of GERD as the underlying cause for patients' symptoms (Fig 3–1). Beedassy et al[6] showed that patients with a positive symptom index were significantly more likely to have an abnormal pH test. Of the 52 patients with chest pain, only 10 had a positive symptom index. Of those, 80% had an abnormal pH study as compared with 36% of the patients with a negative symptom index. However, Dekel et al[7] found that a positive symptom index is a relatively uncommon phenomenon in NCCP patients regardless if GERD is present or absent. This is primarily due to lack of reported chest pain symptoms during the pH study.

Although studies have shown a high association between NCCP and GERD, the mere presence of esophageal inflammation (erosive esophagitis) or abnormal acid exposure suggests association only. In contrast, improvement of chest pain symptoms as a result of antireflux treatment supports causality. Studies have demonstrated that up to 80% of NCCP patients with either erosive esophagitis or abnormal pH testing responded to potent antireflux treatment.[3,8] Consequently, in the presence of esophageal mucosal injury and/or abnormal esophageal acid exposure, it is highly likely that GERD is the underlying cause of patient's symptoms.

In a subgroup of patients with cardiac-related chest pain, acid exposure may play a role in triggering cardiac angina. Both organs share similar sensory innervation. Additionally, acid exposure may reduce coronary blood flow as shown by Chauhan et al.[9] In this study, the investigators evaluated patients with syndrome X

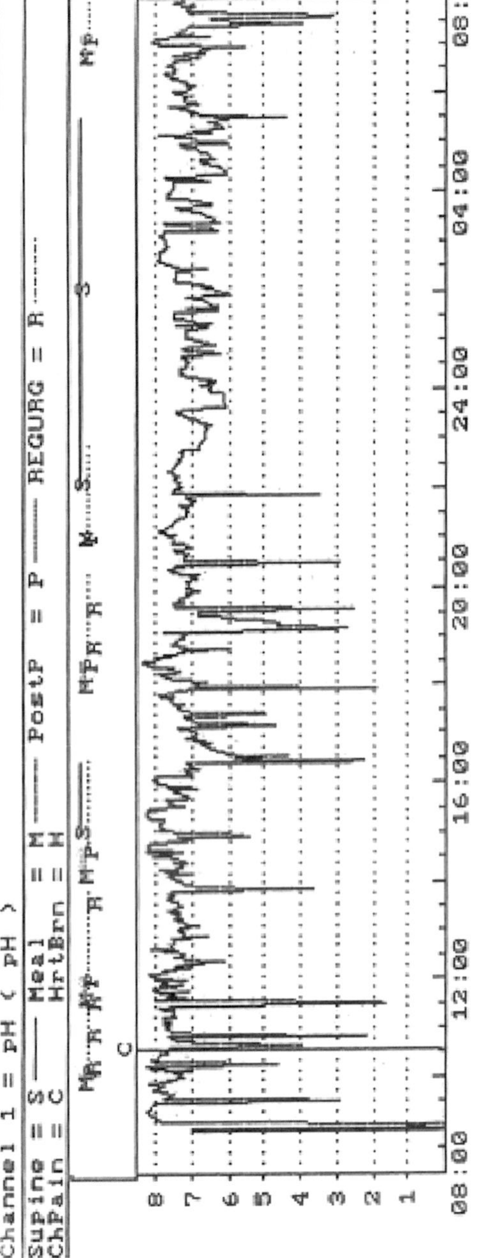

Fig 3–1. A pH testing strip demonstrating a chest pain event (C) that correlated with an acid reflux event in a patient with NCCP.

(negative coronary angiogram but positive stress test) and demonstrated that acidification of the distal esophagus significantly reduced the coronary blood flow resulting in reports of angina.

Acid has also been demonstrated to sensitize esophageal sensory afferents to subsequent mechanical stimuli, such as intraesophageal balloon distension. Further discussion of this topic is presented in the visceral hypersensitivity section.

Esophageal Dysmotility

In NCCP patients who lack any evidence of GERD, esophageal dysmotility is commonly entertained as the underlying cause. However, the role of esophageal motility abnormalities in non-GERD-related NCCP remains to be elucidated. This is primarily due to lack of any relationship between documentation of esophageal dysmotility on manometry and concomitant reports of chest pain. Furthermore, chest pain may be markedly reduced in the absence of any improvement in a patient's esophageal motor disorder.

Only 28% of patients with non-GERD-related NCCP, who underwent esophageal manometry at a tertiary referral center with a major interest in esophageal motility, were found to have an esophageal motility disorder.[10] Similarly, by using the Clinical Outcomes Research Initiative (CORI) database, Dekel et al[11] evaluated 160 NCCP subjects from academic, private, and VA medical centers and demonstrated that only 30% of patients with NCCP had an abnormal esophageal manometry.

The distribution of esophageal motility disorders in patients presenting with non-GERD-related NCCP has scarcely been studied. Figure 3–2 summarizes the two currently available studies that assessed distribution of esophageal motility abnormalities among patients with NCCP. In the study by Dekel et al the most common identified motor disorder was hypotensive LES (61%) followed by hypertensive LES, nonspecific esophageal motility disorder (NEMD), and nutcracker esophagus (10% each). It is likely that more patients with GERD ended up in the Dekel et al study, due to the higher prevalence rate of hypotensive LES. In contrast, Katz et al[10] reported that the most common motor disorder encountered in patients with non-GERD-related NCCP was nutcracker esophagus, followed by nonspecific esophageal motility disorders, diffuse esophageal spasm, hypertensive LES, and achalasia. Regardless, all studies have demonstrated that two-thirds of the patients with non-GERD-related NCCP have normal esophageal motility.

Overall, the finding of a high prevalence of nutcracker esophagus in NCCP patients is common and highly intriguing. Nutcracker esophagus, which is defined manometrically as high-amplitude contractions in the distal esophagus (>180 mm Hg) in the presence of a normally functioning LES, remains an area of intense controversy. Investigators have long argued about the clinical relevance of such a manometric phenomenon.[12] However, Achem et al reported that most patients with chest pain associated with nutcracker esophagus responded symptomatically to antireflux treatment.[13] Normalization of the nutcracker motility phenomenon was documented only in the minority of patients, suggesting that GERD was the likely cause of their symptoms rather than the high amplitude contractions in the distal esophagus. Therefore, esophageal motor disorders

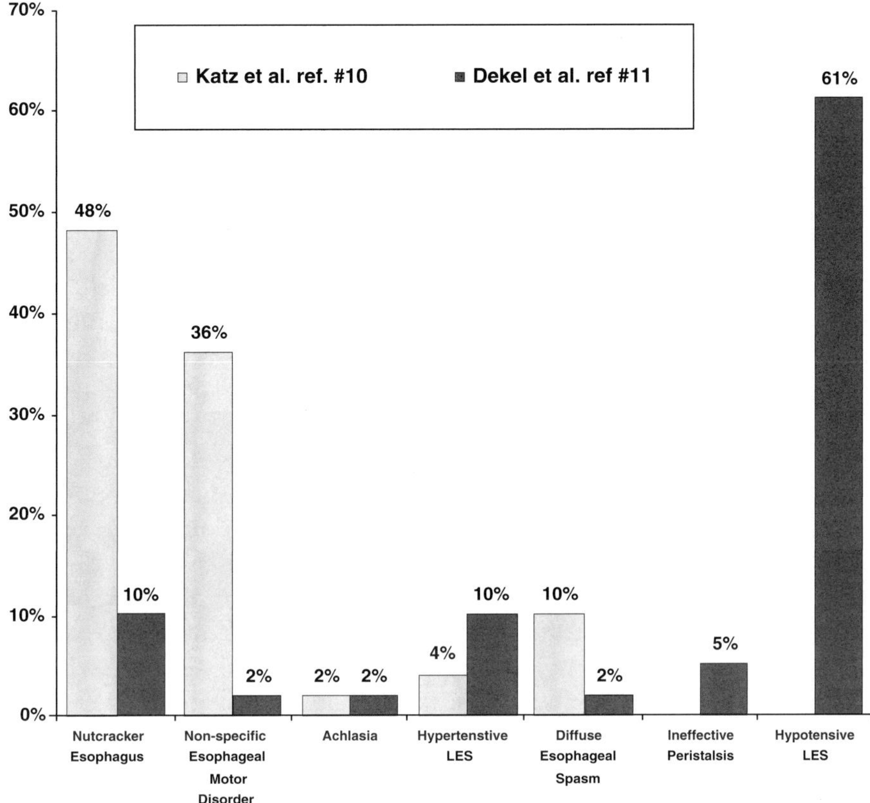

Fig 3–2. Distribution of esophageal motility abnormalities in patients with non-GERD-related NCCP.[10,11]

per se may not be the direct cause of patients' symptoms but may in fact serve as a surrogate marker for esophageal abnormality that is presently poorly understood.[14] Alternatively, esophageal motor disorder in NCCP (except achalasia) may have no etiologic role in symptom generation and thus should not be pursued diagnostically and therapeutically.

High-frequency intraluminal ultrasonography has been introduced as a novel modality to study the relationship between esophageal motor events and symptoms. The technique has been a useful tool for evaluating smooth muscle contractions.[15] The capability of intraluminal ultrasonography to evaluate changes

in the thickness of the longitudinal muscle of the esophagus has been used to determine the relationship between esophageal symptoms and motor changes of the esophageal wall.

Using intraluminal ultrasonography, Balaban and colleagues demonstrated that most chest pain episodes in patients with NCCP were preceded by sustained thickening of the esophageal smooth muscle wall due to longitudinal muscle contraction that was not detected by esophageal manometry catheter.[16] The same muscular changes were noted after edrophonium-induced chest pain. The authors suggested that the duration rather than the magnitude of the longitudinal muscle contraction is the determining factor for generating esophageal pain. In this study, swallow-associated longitudinal muscle contractions lasted an average of 6.4 seconds, whereas contractions associated with chest pain persisted for a mean of 68.0 seconds. Similar studies in patients with GERD revealed that the mean duration of sustained longitudinal muscle contractions during heartburn was 44.9 seconds.[17] The motor changes were also observed in patients who reported heartburn that was unrelated to acid reflux events, further supporting the investigator's hypothesis that this sustained esophageal muscle contraction is responsible for generation of esophageal symptoms, such as chest pain and heartburn.

Even though high-frequency intraluminal ultrasonography has been a valuable research tool to assess the biomechanics of the human esophagus, its exact role in evaluating esophageal related symptoms has not been fully elucidated.[18] Initial studies provided intriguing data, but other investigators have yet to replicate these findings. Furthermore, the technique is highly operator dependent, and interpretation is performed manually. Presently, it is unclear if sustained contractions of the esophageal longitudinal muscle may represent an epiphenomenon that occurs with symptoms rather than being the trigger itself for symptoms.

Visceral Hypersensitivity

The mechanisms of pain in patients with non-GERD-related NCCP are not fully understood. Numerous studies that focused primarily on this group of patients have consistently documented alteration in pain perception regardless of whether esophageal dysmotility was present. The underlying mechanisms for esophageal hypersensitivity in patients with NCCP remain an area of intense research. Peripheral and central sensitization of esophageal sensory afferents and spinal cord neurons has been suggested to result in heightened responses to innocuous and noxious intraesophageal stimuli.[19,20] It has been postulated that inflammation or other injuries to the esophageal mucosa sets off a cascade of events that leads to upregulation of receptors, which, in turn, induces the development of visceral hypersensitivity through peripheral and central sensitization.[20] The presence of esophageal hypersensitivity can be demonstrated long after the original stimulus has disappeared and the mucosa has healed. It is still unclear what factors determine the long-term persistence of esophageal hypersensitivity.

Acute tissue irritation on visceral afferent pathways has been well characterized in the form of peripheral and central sensitization.[5] Such sensitization manifests as increased background activity of sensory neurons, the lowering of nociceptive thresholds, changes in stimulus response curves, and enlargements of receptive fields. During a noxious event, a series of counterregulatory mechanisms are activated that are aimed at containing the development of both the acute and any long-lasting sensitization.[5]

Peripheral sensitization involves the reduction of esophageal pain threshold and an increase in the transduction processes of primary afferent neurons.[21] Esophageal tissue injury, inflammation, spasm, or just repetitive mechanical stimulation can sensitize peripheral afferent nerves.

Several seminal studies, performed during the mid-1980s, were the first to demonstrate that patients with non-GERD-related NCCP demonstrated lower perception thresholds for pain. In the first study, a balloon was positioned 10 cm above the LES and distended in a stepwise fashion using a hand-held syringe. When air was injected (within 2 seconds) in 1-mL increments to a maximum of 10 mL into the balloon attached to a manometry catheter, patients with noncardiac chest pain were more likely to experience pain (18 of 30) than were normal control subjects (6 of 30).[22] In this study, the intraesophageal volume at the onset of pain also distinguished patients from control subjects, with chest pain patients experiencing pain at balloon volumes of less than 8 mL and the few control subjects experiencing pain at volumes of 9 mL or more. A second report evaluating 50 patients with NCCP and 30 healthy volunteers found that 28 (56%) had their "typical" chest pain during balloon inflation as compared to 6 (20%) of the normal controls. Again, most of these patients (24 of 28) had their pain at volumes less than 8 mL.[23] Presence of abnormal motility did not predict a positive test result. When intraballoon pressures were used as a measure of esophageal wall tone, no difference between control subjects and NCCP patients was noted.

Rao et al used impedance planimetry, which consists of a probe with four ring electrodes, three pressure sensors, and a balloon, to evaluate 24 consecutive patients and 12 healthy controls.[24] Stepwise balloon distensions demonstrated lower perception thresholds for first sensation, moderate discomfort, and pain in NCCP patients as compared to normal controls. Typical chest pain was reproduced in 83% of the NCCP patients. In noncardiac chest pain patients, the reac-

tivity of the esophagus to balloon distension was greater, the pressure elastic modulus was higher and the tension-strain association showed that the esophageal wall was less distensible.

Rao et al[25] also performed graded balloon distension of the esophagus using impedance planimetry in 16 consecutive patients with NCCP (normal esophageal evaluation) and 13 healthy control subjects. Patients who experienced chest pain during the balloon distension were subsequently restudied after receiving intravenous atropine. Balloon distensions reproduced chest pain at lower sensory thresholds than controls in most NCCP subjects. Similar findings were documented after atropine administration despite relaxed and more deformable esophageal wall. Thus, the investigators concluded that hyperalgesia, rather than motor dysfunction, is the predominant mechanism for functional chest pain.

Sarkar et al[26] recruited 19 healthy volunteers and 7 patients with NCCP. Hydrochloric acid was infused into the distal esophagus during a period of 30 minutes. Sensory responses to electrical stimulation were monitored within the acid-exposed distal esophagus and the nonexposed proximal esophagus both before and after infusion. In the healthy subjects, acid infusion into the distal esophagus lowered the pain threshold in the upper esophagus. Patients with NCCP already had a lower resting esophageal pain threshold than healthy subjects. After acid perfusion, their pain threshold in the proximal esophagus fell further and for a longer duration than was the case for the healthy subjects. Additionally, there was a decrease in pain threshold after the acid infusion in the anterior chest wall. This study demonstrated the development of secondary allodynia (visceral hypersensitivity to innocuous stimulus in normal tissue that is in proximity to site of tissue injury) in the proximal esophagus by repeated acid exposure of the distal esophagus. The concurrent visceral and somatic pain hypersensitivity is, most likely, caused by central sensitization (increase in excitability of spinal cord neurons induced by activation of nociceptive C-fibers in the area of the tissue injury). The patients with NCCP demonstrated both visceral hypersensitivity and amplified secondary allodynia in the esophagus. However, it is unclear from the study what mechanism is responsible for the exaggerated secondary allodynia and what initiates central sensitization in patients with NCCP. It is interesting to note that other studies[5] on NCCP, using a similar human model of acute tissue irritation by acid infusion, showed no significant effect on pain thresholds.

In one study,[27] healthy subjects underwent perfusion of the distal esophagus with either normal saline or 0.1 N hydrochloric acid. Subsequently, perceptual responses to intraluminal esophageal balloon distention, were evaluated using electronic barostat. As compared with saline, acid perfusion reduced the perception threshold (innocuous sensation) and tended to reduce the pain threshold (aversive sensation). This study demonstrated short-term sensitization of mechanosensitive afferent pathways by transient exposure to acid. The authors suggested that in patients with NCCP, acid reflux induces sensitization of the esophagus that may subsequently alter the way in which the esophagus perceives otherwise normal esophageal distensions.

In a recent study by Sarkar et al,[28] 14 GERD-related NCCP patients and 8 normal controls underwent an esophageal electrical stimulation protocol in the proximal part of the esophagus. The NCCP patients demonstrated lower perception thresholds for pain as compared to the normal control. After 6 weeks of high-dose PPI (omeprazole 20 mg BID), there was an increase in the perception thresholds for pain during electrical stimulation of the proximal part of the esophagus. This is the first study to demonstrate that NCCP patients with evidence of GERD have esophageal hypersensivity that is responsive to PPI therapy.

Abnormal cerebral processing of esophageal stimuli in patients with NCCP has been shown in a study[19] of 12 healthy subjects and 8 patients with NCCP. The aim of the study was to compare cortical-evoked potentials and power spectrum analysis of heart rate variability during electrical esophageal stimulation in patients with NCCP and healthy subjects. Cortical-evoked potentials were recorded using 22 standard electroencephalogram scalp electrodes. Patients with NCCP perceived lower intensities, which were associated with a greater cardiovagal reflex response and decreased sympathetic outflow during electrical esophageal stimulation, than did healthy subjects. Because the cortical-evoked potentials, in response to electrical esophageal stimulation, were smaller in patients with NCCP than in healthy subjects, the authors suggested that the increased perception of esophageal stimuli may result from enhanced cerebral processing of visceral sensory input in patients with NCCP, rather than from hyperalgesic responses in visceral afferent pathways.

Hobson et al explored the neurophysiologic basis of esophageal hypersensitivity in a cohort of NCCP patients.[29] All patients underwent esophageal manometry, esophageal-evoked potentials to electrical stimulation, and pH testing. The authors were able to document three distinct phenotypic classifications of the NCCP group. Subgroup 1 demonstrated normal esophageal-evoked potential latencies with reduced pain thresholds indicative of enhanced afferent transmission and, therefore, increased esophageal afferent pathway sensitivity. Subgroup 2 demonstrated increased esophageal-evoked potential latencies with reduced pain thresholds indicative of normal afferent transmission to the cortex but heightened secondary cortical processing. Subgroup 3 was composed of NCCP patients with normal esophageal-evoked potential latencies and normal pain thresholds.

Several studies have documented altered autonomic function in patients with NCCP. Tougas et al[30] assessed autonomic activity using power spectral analysis of heart rate variability before and after esophageal acidification of patients with NCCP and matched healthy control subjects. Of the patients with NCCP, 68% were considered acid sensitive (developed anginalike symptoms during esophageal acidification). The acid-sensitive patients had a higher baseline heart rate and lower baseline vagal activity than acid-insensitive patients. During acid infusion, vagal cardiac outflow increased in acid-sensitive but not in acid-insensitive patients. The same investigators have already documented an increase in vagal activity in patients with NCCP during other intraesophageal stimuli (mechanical and electrical). Interestingly, in a recent study, the authors found a significant alteration in the autonomic nervous system activity in NCCP patients infected with *Helicobacter pylori* versus NCCP patients who were not infected with the bacteria.[31] The authors

suggested that *Helicobacter pylori* infection may affect autonomic activity in NCCP patients. The role that altered autonomic function plays in the pathogenesis of NCCP remains speculative. As has been stated by Tougas,[32] in most cases in which both central and autonomic factors are involved, it is the effect of the former that most likely leads to the occurrence of the latter.

In addition to cortical-evoked potentials, other techniques have been increasingly used to evaluate brain-gut relationship in patients with esophageal disorders, including those with NCCP. These techniques include positron emission tomography (PET) and functional magnetic resonance imaging (fMRI). The gastrointestinal tract is intricately connected to the central nervous system by pathways that are continuously sampling and modulating gut function.[33]

PET scanning is an established method to study the functional neuroanatomy of the human brain.[34,35] Radio-labeled compounds allow the study of biochemical and physiologic processes involved in cerebral metabolism.[33] Tomographic images represent spatial distribution of radioisotopes in the brain. Regional cerebral blood flow is studied with labeled water ($H_2^{15}O$) and glucose metabolism with ^{18}Fl-labeled fluorodeoxyglucose. Unlike PET, fMRI does not require radioisotopes and hence is considered a safer imaging technique. fMRI detects increases in oxygen concentration in areas of heightened neuronal activity.[35-37] This imaging technique is best suited for locating the site but not the sequence or duration of neuronal activity. Overall, fMRI provides both anatomic and functional information.

Thus far, only a few studies have attempted to assess the cortical process of esophageal sensation in humans. Aziz and colleagues examined the human brain loci involved in the process of esophageal sensation using PET and distal esophageal balloon distension in 8 healthy volunteers.[38] Nonpainful stimuli elicited bilateral activation along the central sulcus, insular cortex, and the frontal and parietal operculum. Painful stimuli resulted in intense activation of the same areas and additional activation of the right anterior insular cortex and anterior cingulated gyrus. The former is important in affective processing whereas the latter is important in pain processing and generating an affective and cognitive response to pain.[39-41] In another study, the same group of investigators evaluated the spatiotemporal correlates of exogenous neural activity evoked by painful esophageal stimulation using recorded magnetoencephalographic (MEG) responses.[42] The study showed that exogenous cortical neural activity evoked by experimental esophageal pain is processed simultaneously in somatosensory and posterior insula regions. Activity in the anterior insula and cingulate—brain regions that process the affective aspects of esophageal pain—occurs significantly later in the somatosensory regions. Sex differences were not observed.

Further studies are needed to assess cerebral activation in patients with different esophageal disorders. In addition, it would be of great interest to determine whether there are differences in central processing of an intraesophageal stimulus in patients with NCCP. It is also important to begin to examine the role of psychophysiologic states such as stress, anxiety, and depression and their effects on central nuclei involved with perception of esophageal stimuli.

Psychological Comorbidity

As with other functional bowel disorders, psychological comorbidity is common in patients with NCCP. In some patients, chest pain is part of a host of symptoms that characterize panic attacks.[43] The symptoms of panic attack are a common cause for emergency room visits for chest pain. In a large study that encompassed 441 consecutive ambulatory patients presenting with chest pain to the emergency department of a heart center, 25% were diagnosed as suffering from a panic attack.[44]

It has been estimated that 17 to 43% of patients with NCCP suffer from a psychological abnormality, primarily anxiety, panic disorder, and hypochondriasis.[45] Song et al[46] evaluated the psychological profiles of 113 patients with chest pain and a variety of esophageal motility abnormalities, 23 symptomatic control subjects (similar symptoms but without esophageal motility abnormalities), and 27 asymptomatic control subjects. All participants were assessed by the Beck Depression Inventory, Spielberger State—Trait Anxiety Inventory, and the psychosomatic symptom checklist. Patients with esophageal symptoms and either hypertensive lower esophageal sphincter, nutcracker esophagus, or hypotensive contractions exhibited increased somatization, anxiety, and depression. Among esophageal symptoms, chest pain was closely correlated with psychometric abnormalities.

Higher ratings on anxiety and depression scales influence pain reporting and may contribute to the psychosocial morbidity suffered by these patients. For example, Lantinga and associates found that patients with noncardiac chest pain had higher levels of neuroticism and psychiatric morbidity before and after cardiac catheterization than did patients with coronary artery disease.[47] This finding appears to have prognostic significance because these patients display less improvement in pain, more frequent pain episodes, greater social maladjustment, and more anxiety disorders at 1-year follow-up than do individuals with relatively low initial levels of psychosocial disturbance.

Summary

Various underlying mechanisms have been described in patients with noncardiac chest pain (NCCP). By far, gastroesophageal reflux disease (GERD) is the most common cause and thus requires initial attention when patients with NCCP are managed. Esophageal dysmotility can be demonstrated in 30% of the NCCP patients but appears to play a very limited role in symptom generation. A significant number of patients with NCCP lack any evidence of GERD and have been consistently shown to have reduced perception thresholds for pain. Peripheral and/or central sensitization has been suggested to be responsible for visceral hypersensitivity in NCCP patients. Further understanding of the underlying mechanisms for pain in patients with NCCP will likely improve our current therapeutic approach.

References

1. Locke G, 3rd, Talley NJ, Fett SL, Zinsmeister AR, Melton LJ, 3rd. Prevalence and clinical spectrum of gastroesophageal reflux: a population-based study in Olmstead County, Minnesota. *Gastroenterology.* 1997;112(5):1448-1456.

2. Eslick GD. Noncardiac chest pain: epidemiology, natural history, health care seeking, and quality of life. *Gastroenterol Clin North Am.* 2004;33(1):1-23.

3. Fass R, Fennerty MB, Ofman JJ, et al. The clinical and economic value of a short course of omeprazole patients with noncardiac chest pain. *Gastroenterology.* 1998;115(1):42-49.

4. Fass R, Winters GF. Evaluation of the patient with noncardiac chest pain: is gastroesophageal reflux disease or an esophageal motility disorder the cause? *Medscape Gastroenterol J.* 2001;3(6):1-7.

5. Fass R, Naliboff B, Higa L, et al. Differential effect of long-term esophageal acid exposure on mechanosensitivity and chemosensitivity in humans. *Gastroenterology.* 1998;115(6):1363-1373.

6. Beedassy A, Katz PO, Gruber A, Peghini PL, Castell DO. Prior sensitization of esophageal mucosa by acid reflux predisposes to reflux-induced chest pain. *J Clin Gastroenterol.* 2000;31(2):121-124.

7. Dekel R, Martinez-Hawthorne SD, Guillen RJ, Fass R. Evaluation of symptom index in identifying gastroesophageal reflux disease-related noncardiac chest pain. *J Clin Gastroenterol.* 2004;38(1):24-29.

8. Fass R, Fennerty MB, Johnson C, Camargo L, Sampliner RE. Correlation of ambulatory 24-hour esophageal pH monitoring results with symptom improvement in patients with noncardiac chest pain due to gastroesophageal reflux disease. *J Clin Gastroenterol.* 1999;28(1):36-39.

9. Chauhan A, Petch MC, Schofield PM. Cardio-oesophageal reflex in humans as a mechanism for "linked angina." *Eur Heart J.* 1996;17(3):407-413.

10. Katz PO, Dalton CB, Richter JE, Wu WC, Castell DO. Esophageal testing of patients with noncardiac chest pain or dysphagia. Results of three years' experi-

ence in 1161 patients. *Ann Intern Med.* 1987;106(4):593-597.

11. Dekel R, Pearson T, Wendel C, De Garmo P, Fennerty MB, Fass R. Assessment of oesophageal motor function in patients with dysphagia or chest pain—the Clinical Outcomes Research Initiative experience. *Aliment Pharmacol Ther.* 2003; 18(11-12):1083-1089.

12. Kahrilas PJ. Editorial: Nutcracker esophagus: an idea whose time has gone? *Am J Gastroenterol.* 1993;88(2):167-169.

13. Achem SR, Kolts BE, Wears R, Burton L, Richter JE. Chest pain associated with nutcracker esophagus: a preliminary study of the role of gastroesophageal reflux. *Am J Gastroenterol.* 1993;88(2):187-192.

14. Richter JE. Oesophageal motility disorders. *Lancet.* 2001;358(9284):823-828.

15. Nguyen HN, Silney J, Matern S. Multiple intraluminal electrical impedancometry for recording of upper gastrointestinal motility: current results and further implications. *Am J Gastroenterol.* 1999;94(2):306-317.

16. Balaban DH, Yamamoto Y, Liu J, et al. Sustained esophageal contraction: a marker of esophageal chest pain identified by intraluminal ultrasonography. *Gastroenterology.* 1999;116(1):29-37.

17. Pehlivanov N, Liu J, Mittal RK. Sustained esophageal contraction: a motor correlate of heartburn symptoms. *Am J Physiol Gastrointest Liver Physiol.* 2001;281(3): G743-G751.

18. Takeda T, Kassab G, Liu J, Puckett JL, Mittal RR, Mittal RK. A novel ultrasound technique to study the biomechanics of the human esophagus in vivo. *Am J Physiol Gastrointest Liver Physiol.* 2002; 282(5):G785-G793.

19. Hollerbach S, Bulat R, May A, et al. Abnormal cerebral processing oesophageal stimuli in patients with noncardiac chest pain (NCCP). *Neurogastroenterol Motil.* 2000;12(6):555-565.

20. Aziz Q. Acid sensors in the gut: a taste of things to come. *Eur J Gastroenterol Hepatol.* 2001;13(8):885-888.

21. Handwerker HO, Reeh PW. Nociceptors: chemosensitivity and sensitization by chemical agents. In: Willis WD, Jr., ed. *Hyperalgesia and Allodynia.* New York, NY: Raven Press; 1992:107.

22. Richter JE, Barish CF, Castell DO. Abnormal sensory perception in patients with esophageal chest pain. *Gastroenterology.* 1986;91(4):845-852.

23. Barish CF, Castell DO, Richter JE. Graded esophageal balloon distention. A new provocative test for noncardiac chest pain. *Dig Dis Sci.* 1986;31(12):1292-1298.

24. Rao SS, Gregersen H, Hayek B, Summers RW, Christensen J. Unexplained chest pain: the hypersensitive, hyperreactive, and poorly compliant esophagus. *Ann Intern Med.* 1996;124(11):950-958.

25. Rao SS, Hayek B, Summers RW. Functional chest pain of esophageal origin: hyperalgesia or motor dysfunction. *Am J Gastroenterol.* 2001;96(9):2584-2589.

26. Sarkar S, Aziz Q, Woolf CJ, Hobson AR, Thompson DG. Contribution of central sensitisation to the development of non-cardiac chest pain. *Lancet.* 2000; 356(9236):1154-1159.

27. Hu WH, Martin CJ, Talley NJ. Intraesophageal acid perfusion sensitizes the esophagus to mechanical distension: a Barostat study. *Am J Gastroenterol.* 2000;95(9): 2189-2194.

28. Sarkar S, Thompson DG, Woolf CJ, Hobson AR, Millane T, Aziz Q. Patients with chest pain and occult gastroesophageal reflux demonstrate visceral pain hypersensitivity which may be partially responsive to acid suppression. *Am J Gastroenterol.* 2004;99(10):1998-2006.

29. Hobson A, Furlong P, Sarkar S, et al. Neurophysiologic assessment of esophageal sensory processing in noncardiac chest pain. *Gastroenterol.* 2006;130:80-88.

30. Tougas G, Spaziani R, Hollerbach S, et al. Cardiac autonomic function and oesophageal acid sensitivity in patients with non-cardiac chest pain. *Gut.* 2001;49(5): 706-712.

31. Budzynski J, Klopocka M, Bujak R, Swiatkowski M, Pulkowski G, Sinkiewicz W. Autonomic nervous function in *Helicobacter pylori*-infected patients with atypical chest pain studied by analysis of heart rate variability. *Eur J Gastroenterol Hepatol.* 2004;16:451-457.

32. Tougas G. The autonomic nervous system in functional bowel disorders. *Gut.* 2000;47(suppl 4):iv78-80.

33. Aziz Q, Thompson DG. Brain-gut axis in health and disease. *Gastroenterology.* 1998;114(3):559-578.

34. Hartshorne MF. Positron emission tomography. In: Orrison WW, Lewine JD, Sanders JA, Hartshorne MF, eds. *Functional Brain Imaging.* St. Louis, Mo: Mosby-Year Book; 1995:187-212.

35. Aine CJ. A conceptual overview and critique of functional neuroimaging techniques in humans: I. MRI/FMRI and PET. *Crit Rev Neurobiol.* 1995;9(2-3):229-309.

36. Smout AJPM, DeVore MS, Dalton CB, Castell DO. Cerebral potentials evoked by oesophageal distension in patients with non-cardiac chest pain. *Gut.* 1992; 33(3):298-302.

37. Sanders JA, Orrison WW. Functional magnetic resonance imaging. In: Orrison WW, Lewine JD, Sanders JA, Hartshorne MF, eds. *Functional Brain Imaging.* St. Louis, Mo: Mosby-Year Book; 1995: 239-326.

38. Aziz Q, Andersson JL, Valind S, et al. Identification of human brain loci processing esophageal sensation using positron emission tomography. *Gastroenterology.* 1997;113(1):50-59.

39. Minshohima S, Morrow TJ, Koeppe RA. Involvement of insular cortex in central autonomic regulation during painful thermal stimulation. *J Cereb Blood Flow Metab.* 1995;15(suppl 1):1355-1358.

40. Talbot JD, Marrett S, Evans AC, Meyer E, Bushnell MC, Duncan GH. Multiple representations of pain in human cerebral cortex. *Science.* 1991;251(4999):1355-1358.

41. Vogt BA, Sikes RW, Vogt LJ. Anterior cingulate cortex and the medial pain system. In: Vogt BA, Gabriel M, eds. *Neurobiology of Cingulate Cortex and Limbic Thalamus.* Boston: Birkhauser; 1994:313-344.

42. Hobson A, Furlong P, Worthen S, et al. Real-time imaging of human cortical activity evoked by painful esophageal stimulation. *Gastroenterol.* 2005;128:610-619.

43. Potokar JP, Nutt DJ. Chest pain: panic attack or heart attack? *Int J Clin Pract.* 2000;54(2):110-114.

44. Fleet RP, Dupuis G, Marchand A, Burelle D, Arsenault A, Beitman BD. Panic disorder in emergency department chest pain patients: prevalence, comorbidity, suicidal ideation, and physician recognition. *Am J Med.* 1996;101(4):371-380.

45. van Peski-Oosterbaan AS, Spinhoven P, van Rood Y, van der Does JW, Bruschke AV, Rooijmans HG. Cognitive-behavioral therapy for noncardiac chest pain: a randomized trial. *Am J Med.* 2000;106(4): 424-429.

46. Song CW, Lee SJ, Jeem YT, et al. Inconsistent association of esophageal symptoms, psychometric abnormalities and dysmotility. *Am J Gastroenterol.* 2001;96(8): 2312-2316.

47. Lantinga LJ, Sprafkin RP, McCroskery JH, Baker MT, Warner RA, Hill NE. One-year psychosocial follow-up of patients with chest pain and angiographically normal coronary arteries. *Am J Cardiol.* 1988; 62(4):209-213.

CHAPTER 4

Noncardiac, Nonesophageal Causes of Chest Pain

Sami R. Achem
Kenneth R. DeVault

Introduction

The approach to patients with chest pain has continued to evolve over the past several years. Cardiac disease must be excluded as noted elsewhere in this book, but even in patients referred to cardiologists, up to 50% will ultimately be found to have no evidence of cardiac disease. In a large survey of primary care providers, it was found that after a cardiac etiology has been excluded, esophageal causes are often addressed as the next most likely etiology for pain.[1] These physicians offered patients a trial of proton-pump inhibitors as their preferred approach, but they obviously consider other noncardiac, nonesophageal disorders as important, as the next most common test ordered was a chest x-ray. This test is done to exclude conditions such as pneumonia, rib fracture, pneumothorax, and congestive heart failure.[2] They were also more likely to do a CT scan of the chest than an esophageal manometry or pH test and felt that musculoskeletal and psychiatric etiologies were the next most common after the esophagus. The site of the patient encounter seems to be a very important factor in the proportion of patients with a given etiology for their pain. In recent studies, primary care offices found musculoskeletal pain to be responsible for chest pain in 36% of patients and cardiac causes to be present in 16% where patient presenting to emergency units were much less likely to have musculoskeletal problems (7%) and much more likely to have cardiac disease (54%).[3,4]

In this chapter we address potential causes for chest pain that do not directly involve the heart and esophagus (Table 4–1).

Table 4–1. Common Noncardiac, Nonesophageal Etiologies for Chest Pain

1. Musculoskeletal
   a. Tietze's syndrome
   b. Costochrondritis
   c. Fibromyalgia
   d. Precordial catch syndrome
   e. Slipping rib syndrome
2. Gastrointestinal
   a. Gastric
   b. Biliary tree
   c. Pancreatic
   d. Intra-abdominal masses (benign and malignant)
3. Pulmonary
   a. Pneumonia
   b. Pulmonary embolus
   c. Lung cancer
   d. Sarcoidosis
   e. Pneumothorax and pneumomediastinum
   f. Pleural effusions
   g. Intrathoracic masses (benign and malignant)
4. Miscellaneous
   a. Aortic disorders
   b. Pericarditis and myocarditis
   c. Pulmonary hypertension
   d. Herpes zoster
   e. Drug-induced pain
   f. Sickle cell crisis
   g. Psychological disorders

Musculoskeletal

Most investigators agree that, following negative cardiac and pulmonary evaluations, referral to a gastroenterologist is commonly considered in patients with unexplained chest pain. However, pain arising from musculoskeletal (MSK) sources, rather than esophageal or gastrointestinal visceral pain, may account for the patient's pain. Gastroenterologists may not be as familiar with the many sources of chest pain (CP) originating from the thoracic cage or myofascial sources. To compound the problem, there is a paucity of data in the gastroenterological literature focusing on MSK causes of chest pain. In fact, many of these patients may be seen in rheumatology practices,[5] orthopedic practices,[6] pain clinics, or by physical medicine and rehabilitation specialists. CP may originate from disorders affecting the structures of the anterior chest wall, such as the ribs and sternum, or be referred from neck, shoulders, or back. In this section, we review some of the most common and important causes of CP from MSK sources.

Epidemiology

The concern that CP may originate from musculoskeletal sources is not new. Travell and Rinzler in 1948 suggested that pain arising from chest muscles resembled that of angina.[7] In 1950, Allison reported on 50 consecutive patients to which "the diagnosis of coronary artery disease had been wrongfully applied and each case it was found in structures of the chest wall."[8] Although these studies were done prior to the advent of coronary angiography (not available until the 1960s), they indicate that despite the lack of a gold standard to exclude coronary artery disease, clinicians long suspected the role of MSK conditions as imitators of cardiac pain.

The epidemiology of chest wall pain presenting as anginalike CP has been addressed in a series of more contemporary investigations using coronary angiography as the gold standard to exclude heart disease. In the largest epidemiologic study available, investigators from Sweden evaluated more than 7,000 patients seen in an emergency department for suspected MI and noted that 26% of patients had MSK causes of CP.[9] Levine and Mascette suggested that MSK causes of CP were present in 11 to 66% of 67 patients undergoing cardiac evaluation. They described reproduction of chest wall tenderness in 11% and nonreproducing chest wall tenderness in 61% of their patients.[10] Husser et al studied 37 consecutive patients with CP and normal coronary arteries. Six (15%) were reported to have MSK sources of chest pain (four costochondritis, one vertebral pain, and one fibromyalgia). Half of these patients also were diagnosed with coexisting gastroesophageal reflux.[11] Wise et al evaluated 100 consecutive patients with CP and negative coronary angiography for chest wall tenderness. A total of 69 had chest wall tenderness, typical pain reproducing patient's chest pain occurred in 16, and 5 patients were diagnosed with fibrositis. None of 25 control subjects (rheumatoid arthritis, osteoarthritis) experienced chest wall tenderness.[12] Ho et al performed a prospective study of 71 patients with CP to examine the prevalence of fibromyalgia (FM).[13] The diagnostic criteria for FM was based on the American Rheumatology Association published guidelines.[14] Subjects were divided in two groups based on the presence ($n = 36$) or absence ($n = 35$) of significant coronary artery disease (CAD). Seven patients (25%) (6 of 7 female) without CAD and 1 patient (male) (3%) with CAD had chest wall tenderness fulfilling criteria for fibromyalgia. The authors concluded that fibromyalgia is more common among women with anginalike pain and insignificant degrees of

CAD. Mukerji et al evaluated 40 consecutive patients with chest pain and normal coronaries finding that 30% suffered from FM and 10% from costochrondritis, whereas in a group of 40 controls with coronary artery disease only one patient had FM.[15]

A survey of 109 primary clinicians in 37 practices in 18 states and 3 Canadian provinces reported the prevalence of CP diagnosis in primary care offices. In this group of 832 patients, chest wall pain occurred in 65% and costochondritis in 83% (with significant overlap).[16] The specific characteristics of chest pain required for entry and the extent of cardiac investigations the patients underwent were not standardized in this study. Despite those limitations, these findings from a group of primary care providers underscore the high prevalence of MSK in this clinical setting. Similar findings were noted in a prospective study of an established primary care research network over a 12-month period which surveyed 396 patients from academic and nonacademic sites. They found that MSK accounted for 20% of the CP, costochondritis for 13%, gastroesophageal reflux in 13% and "esophageal spasm" in only 4%.[17] Finally, of 407 children with "ill-defined chest pain" admitted to an emergency room (47% had ECG and 34% echocardiograms); MSK causes of chest pain were reported in 15%.[18]

There are a number of concerns with the studies reviewed in previous paragraphs. Most of the studies have a relatively small sample size and some fail to define the basis for the diagnostic criteria of MSK. The lack of a diagnostic gold standard or an objective test that can be applied to establish unequivocally the source of pain begs the question whether findings such as "chest wall tenderness" explain the patient's pain. Until an objective diagnostic test is developed, only longitudinal follow-up may establish the consistency of the diagnosis and whether pain resolves following therapy aimed at myofascial pain. Despite those limitations, the studies reviewed indicate that, by all accounts, MSK sources of chest pain are common in patients with CP in adult, pediatric, emergency medicine, or office-based practices.

General Clinical Features

As there is no conclusive diagnostic test for MSK, the diagnosis of CP arising from MSK origins rests on a careful history and physical examination. The following general features should alert the physician about the possible origin of MSK pain. The onset of the pain is often insidious. There may be a history of trauma or unusual physical activity. The pain is often localized to the affected side but may radiate widely. Increase of pain with movement and amelioration with heat, analgesics, or local infiltration are additional features. Nocturnal pain is uncommon. On examination, persistent local tenderness is the dominant feature of MSK disorders. Reproduction of the patient's pain on palpation may also be noted. Focal swelling may be an additional feature.[19] We now cover several of the specific MSK causes of CP.

Tietze's Syndrome

Alexander Tietze first described this syndrome in 1921.[20] Tietze's syndrome is a rare disorder, characterized by tender, non-suppurative swelling of the costochondral cartilages in the upper costosternal region.[21] The age of onset is usually before 40, and both sexes are affected equally. There is no occupational, racial, or geographic predisposition. The syndrome is usually self-limited and the cause is unknown but a traumatic pathogenesis has been suspected. In most patients, only one joint is involved, usually the second or third costochondral joint but may also include the sternoclavicular joint.[22] The onset of anterior chest pain may be sudden or gradual. The pain may radiate to the arms or shoulders and is aggravated by sneezing, coughing, deep inspiration, lying prone, or twisting motions of the chest. There may be an antecedent history of excessive coughing. The affected cartilage is tender and swollen but there is no heat and erythema. The diagnosis is primarily based on clinical findings. A small study from Italy ($n = 4$ patients) found that ultrasound or computed tomography imaging of the chest was helpful in finding "thickened cartilage, inhomogeneous increased echogenicity ($n = 4$) and blurred outline ($n = 3$)." CT showed thickened cartilage and blurred outline ($n = 3$); none of 10 controls showed those signs.[23] This study awaits further confirmation. A small series found that bone scanning failed to be of diagnostic utility.[24] The clinician should also be aware that, occasionally, Tiezte's syndrome may be a manifestation of a neoplasm. A number of small reports have described patients with Tiezte's syndrome who were found to have squamous cell carcinoma of the mediastinum unknown primary site invading the sternum and anterior chest wall,[25] or lymphomas.[26] Treatment involves local heat, analgesics (non-steroidal anti-inflammatory agents) (NSAIDS). For nonresponsive patients local steroid-lidocaine and or intercostal nerve block may be required.[27]

Costochondritis

Costochondritis is a common and poorly understood disorder. It has been given several names: "anterior chest wall syndrome," "parasternal chondrodynia," "costosternal syndrome." A prevalence of 30% has been described among patients presenting for evaluation to the emergency room. In this condition, the second to the fifth costal cartilages are the areas most commonly involved and there is no associated swelling. The disorder typically affects patients older than 40 and usually has a self-limited course but recurrences up to a year have been described. The etiology is undetermined. A possible inflammatory mechanism has been postulated, as patients may show a high erythrocyte sedimentation rate and morning stiffness.[28] The diagnosis is based on a history of anterior chest wall tenderness localized to the chostochondral junction of one or more ribs, without local inflammatory reaction (heat, erythema). Pain can be precipitated during physical exam by: (a) extension of cervical spine and traction of the posterior extended arms, and/or (b) traction of the adducted arm with the head rotated to the ipsilateral side. Tietze's syndrome and costochondritis are not synonymous—the former features costochondral cartilage swelling (costochondritis does not). In a study of 20 patients with costochondritis compared to 10 control subjects with cancer who did not have clinical signs of costochondritis (bone imaging showed no metastasis in all cases), bone scans with 99mTc-methylene diphosphonate were found unhelpful in making the diagnosis of costochondritis.[29] In a study of 25 patients with CP, Freeston et al found that after patients were properly diagnosed, the number of chest pain admissions, hospitalization days, and clinical tests were significantly reduced.[30] Treatment is similar to that prescribed for Tietze's syndrome.

Fibromyalgia

Fibromyalgia (FM), fibrositis, or myofascial syndrome is a chronic disorder characterized by diffuse musculoskeletal pain associated with multiple discrete tender points. FM is a common disorder second in prevalence among rheumatologic conditions only to osteoarthritis.[31] The overall prevalence of fibromyalgia is 0.5 to 5% in the general population but may be up to 15.7% in symptomatic groups.[32] CP has been reported in patients with FM.[33] In 1990, the American College of Rheumatology proposed that a history of chronic, widespread pain and the finding of 11 of 18 possible tender points on exam as the basis for the diagnosis,[14] although a recent paper questioned the acceptance of these criteria.[34] The most accepted suggestive features include: (1) diffuse widespread MSK aching pain and stiffness, particularly in neck, shoulder, chest, and periscapular wall for 3 months; (2) pain that is affected by changes in weather, physical activity, fatigue, and psychological factors; (3) multiple fibrositic tender points at specified sites. (4) nonrestorative sleep, fatigue, and morning stiffness; (5) frequent association with anxiety, depression, irritable bowel syndrome, chronic fatigue, or chronic headache; and (6) normal lab tests and exclusion of other systemic disorders. As the diagnosis of FM rests primarily on clinical grounds, the physician must exclude other clinical conditions such as systemic lupus, rheumatoid arthritis, polymyalgia rheumatica, thyroid, parathyroid disease, malignancy, hepatitis C, and Lyme disease. In addition, FM may coexist with some of those disorders.[35]

FM is part of the family of functional somatic syndromes including irritable bowel syndrome, chronic fatigue syndrome, chronic migraine, low back pain, and irritable bladder. Many patients suffer from various degrees of anxiety, fear, and depression; they often resist efforts to reassure them about the benign nature of the pain. This disorder commonly starts in the third or fourth decade and is five times more common in women. Data suggest a familiar tendency to develop this disorder.[36] Exposure to physical, environmental or emotional "stressors" may precipitate the initiation of symptoms.[37] The etiology and pathogenesis is poorly understood. Increasing evidence points toward nociceptive input from musculoskeletal sources that might either initiate or maintain central sensitization or both. Once central sensitization has been established, only minimal nociceptive input is required for the maintenance of the chronic pain state.[38] Interestingly, Maresca et al studied 22 patients with documented mitral valve prolapse (MVP) where 86% had myofascial chest pain consistent with fibromyalgia.[39]

No drug has been approved for the specific treatment of FM, but tricyclics, dual reuptake inhibitors, anticonvulsants and nonpharmacologic therapies (eg, aerobic exercise) that are known to increase antinociceptive or decrease pronociceptive influences have been tried. Emerging therapies, such as the antidepressants duloxetine and milnacipran and the antiepileptic pregabalin, may offer some efficacy. Cognitive behavioral therapy (CBT) provided worthwhile improvements in pain-related behavior, self-efficacy, coping strategies, and overall physical function in fibromyalgia. Sustained improvements in pain were most consistent when individualized CBT was used to treat patients with juvenile fibromyalgia.[40]

Precordial Catch Syndrome (chest wall twinge or Texidor's twinge)

This is a common self-limited cause of chest pain seen mostly in young children or adolescents. Miller and Texidor first described the syndrome in 1955.[41] They characterized the condition as sudden onset, sharp, stabbing, well-localized precordial pain in 10 patients, one of whom was Miller himself. Later authors coined the phrase Texidor's twinge. The pain has also been described as a "stitch" or "catch." Pain typically occurs at rest, is exacerbated by breathing, is fleeting in nature, lasting 30 seconds to 3 minutes, with sudden and complete resolution. There are no associated symptoms or physical findings.[42] The etiology and pathogenesis are not well understood. Reassurance and conservative therapy is usually the best treatment approach.

Slipping Rib Syndrome

The slipping rib syndrome is a commonly overlooked cause of CP or upper abdominal pain. This disorder was first recognized in 1919 by Cyriax[43] and Davis-Colley coined the term of its current designation in 1922.[44] It has been estimated to occur in 1 to 5% of all causes of consultations in a general medical practice.[45] In 1993, Scott and Scott reported a prevalence of 3% to a general medical/gastroenterology clinic.[46] Despite the fact that this syndrome may occur more frequently than recognized, only 30 papers were found on a computerized search of the literature using specifically the term "slipped rib." The characteristic patient experiences a traumatic injury to the chest wall, frequently during sports. Peterson and Cavanaugh describe an illustrative case of a 14-year-old child experiencing a football injury (helmet tackled) who eluded medical diagnosis for 2 years.[47]

Although the syndrome is usually precipitated by trauma, patients may not always recall a history of trauma. This disorder is thought to arise from the inadequacy or rupture of the interchondral fibrous attachments of the anterior ribs. This disruption allows the costal cartilage tips to sublux, impinging on the intercostal nerves. In most cases there is luxation of the costal cartilage at the 8th, 9th, or 10th ribs. Loosening of the fibrous attachment binding of the lower costal cartilages to one another facilitates a rib tip to curl upward and override the inner aspect of the rib above. Intermittent unilateral pain in the anterior ends of the costal cartilages is the chief complaint. Patients may exacerbate their pain with certain movements such as respiration, or movements of the thorax or extremities. They may also describe a sensation of popping, snapping, clicking, or giving way. On exam, the pain can be duplicated by the "hooking maneuver," first described by Heinz and Zavala in 1977, which consists of curving the examiners fingers under the anterior costal margin and pulling the rib cage anteriorly and superiorly inducing a gentle subluaxation of the affected cartilage.[48] This maneuver may also trigger a palpable click. Three treatment modalities have been proposed: (1) reassurance and explanation; (2) local anesthetic nerve block once or several times; and finally, if all conservative measures fail, (3) excision of the anterior end of the rib and costal margin.

Miscellaneous Musculoskeletal Etiologies

Cervicothoracic pain has been linked to pectoral muscle girdle fatigue. Ryan described that a pure drag on the arm can trigger chest pain. The muscles involved are the elevators of the scapula, the upper part of the trapeziums, and levator scapulas. He reported pain in 75 women associated with chronic drag from bra strap pressure due to breast weight, breast feeding (with the baby carried on the forearm), wearing heavy shoulder bags, regular carrying of market bags.[49] Thoracic disk herniation can also cause CP. In a retrospective review of 55 patients documented by magnetic resonance imaging, 67% presented with "bandlike" chest pain. In this study, 27% underwent surgery, with lesions at or below T9 level more likely to require intervention with good outcome and resolution of symptoms.[50] There are a number of other MSK conditions that can result in CP. They include disorders such as ankylosing spondylitis, intercostal neuralgia, spinal stenosis, metastatic or primary neoplastic disease involving spine or chest wall, and diffuse idiopathic skeletal hyperostosis (DISH) among others.

Gastrointestinal

Gastric Causes

Gastric disorders usually present with pain in the epigastric region, but some patients can interpret this as chest pain. In an interesting pediatric series, the sign of epigastric tenderness was very specific for a GI etiology in patients with a primary symptom of chest pain,[51] but this has not been addressed as extensively in adults. The pain of a peptic ulcer usually varies somewhat throughout the day and if it becomes constant and severe, a complication such as posterior perforation should be considered. Complicated peptic ulcers producing stenosis in the distal stomach usually present with vomiting, but on occasion can produce a syndrome more consistent with gastroesophageal reflux and may cause chest pain. Hiatal hernias can produce pain either from the hernia itself or more likely from diaphragmatic irritation. Severe pain coming from a hernia is suggestive of a complication rather than the hernia itself.[52,53] Gastric volvulus has been reported to produce pain that is very similar to cardiac disease.[54] Laparoscopic gastric banding is a new technique for control of obesity and has been reported to produce chest pain in at least four cases.[55] In this series all patients recovered, but other more serious complications have been reported including mediastinal emphysema[56] and gastric necrosis.[57]

Gallstones and Other Biliary Problems

Problems with the gallbladder and biliary tree usually present with upper abdominal discomfort, although chest and particularly right shoulder pain are also common. The pain of cholelithiasis is typically somewhat vague and episodic whereas persistent pain, especially if accompanied by fever and leukocytosis, is suggestive of cholecystitis or cholangitis.[58] Diagnosis is made clinically with confirmation by ultrasound or other imaging modalities.

Pancreatitis

Pancreatitis also usually presents with upper abdominal pain, but chest pain occurs in some patients. Pain may vary from a mild and tolerable discomfort to severe, constant pain that requires narcotics for relief. Painful pleural and pericardial effusions can complicate this disorder as well. Diagnosis depends upon clinical suspicion followed by laboratory and radiographic confirmation. An early CT scan is particularly helpful in that it may be diagnostic and provide prognostic information.[59]

Other Intra-abdominal Causes

Any process within the abdominal cavity can produce chest pain, particularly if it is in the upper abdomen. Reported examples include; renal hemorrhage,[60] splenic infarction, mesenteric ischemia, and bleeding from a gastric artery.[61]

Pulmonary

As noted above, most primary care providers consider a chest x-ray (CXR) an important early test in noncardiac chest pain, although there are no data reporting the utility of this approach in patients without other specific or at least suggestive pulmonary symptoms. The role of CT scanning in chest pain patients has not been well defined, but these studies are frequently obtained in both acute and chronic pain patients. In a study based in emergency units, 14.2% of patients presenting with chest pain were found to have a pulmonary etiology for their pain.[62] Is this series of unselected patients, pulmonary disease was actually much more common than gastroesophageal disorders (2.4%). Some of the causes of pulmonary disease included pneumonia, spontaneous pneumothorax, pulmonary embolus, and pleuritis.

Pneumonia

Pneumonia is very common with 4 to 6 million cases reported on a yearly basis.[63] Patients with pneumonia typically present with fever and a productive cough. Chest pain has been reported in up to 30% of cases and is usually pleuritic in character.[64] Isolated chest pain without other symptoms more suggestive of infection is probably quite rare. Although the usual pain associated with pneumonia tends to be pleuritic, more severe and constant pain could suggest a complication such as abscess development, cavitation, or extension into the adjacent structures. Pneumonia is usually diagnosed by history, physical examination, and CXR, with only selected cases requiring CT for confirmation or clarification. There are no radiologic features that can be used to distinguish between bacterial, viral, and fungal etiologies.[65] Tuberculosis, especially if cavitating, can present with chest pain as the predominant symptom as can acute histoplasmosis infection.[66,67] The CXR may be falsely negative in pneumonia patients with significant degrees of dehydration and should be repeated after hydration if the diagnosis remains a concern. Rarely, one of the more chronic pulmonary disorders like bronchiolitis obliterans can present with chest pain, although the patient will usually have substantial dyspnea.[68]

Pulmonary Embolus

Pulmonary embolus (PE) has an incidence of greater than 1 per 1,000 and causes up to 100,000 deaths per year in the United States.[69] Chest pain is commonly present and PE must be considered in the differential diagnosis of all CP patients.[70] Whereas PE is a very common diagnosis, most chest pain series actually report a fairly low prevalence. For example, in a coronary care unit where 175 consecutive patients were evaluated, PE was only found in 5 cases.[71] In addition, a Swedish study of over 7,000 emergency department patients with chest pain only found a PE in 0.8%.[72] The classical presentation of chest pain, dyspnea, and hemoptysis is only present in 20% of patients. Clinical suspicion in all patients with acute chest pain is important as only 30% of PEs are diagnosed prior to death.[73] Conversely, fewer than 35% of patients suspected of having PE actually have the diagnosis.[74] Some, but not all, patients will have evidence of peripheral deep venous thrombosis.[75] Recently, D-dimer testing has been advocated as a screening tool where, in patients with a fairly low clinical suspicion of PE, a normal D-dimer level rules out PE with a 99.5% negative predictive value.[76] CT pulmonary angiography has rapidly replaced ventilation perfusion scanning as the primary method used to evaluate for PE. Invasive angiography is rarely performed for diagnosis, but is important in patients with severe disease as it offers the opportunity for intervention (clot removal). The degree of vascular obstruction and underlying comorbidity tend to predict which patients have a simple PE, pulmonary infarction, circulatory collapse, or death.[77]

Lung Cancer

Isolated chest pain is unusual in malignant disease of the pulmonary system, just as in many of the other pulmonary conditions. Some patients will have pain associated with their other more typical symptoms and patients rarely will have isolated dull pain on the side of their lesion. More severe or persistent pain is indicative of invasion of the chest wall or other structures.[78]

Sarcoidosis

Chest pain is common in patients with pulmonary sarcoidosis, although cough and dyspnea are usually present as well. This can occur with isolated pulmonary sarcoid, although it is probably more common in patients with more extensive nodal disease. Sacoidosis can present in several ways. There is an acute or subacute form, which develops abruptly over a period of a few weeks and is associated with constitutional symptoms such as fever, fatigue, malaise, and a vague retrosternal discomfort.[79] The more common form is insidious, developing over a period of months, and is more likely to be associated with isolated pulmonary symptoms. Pleural effusions and rarely pneumo- or hydrothorax may complicate sarcoidosis.

Pneumothorax and Pneumomediastinum

Spontaneous pneumothorax occurs in the absence of trauma and is most commonly caused by apical blebs.[80] This problem should be considered high in the differential diagnosis of a young patient presenting with chest pain, particularly if they are also short of breath. Recurrent pneumothorax occurs in up to 50% of patients in whom the earlier event has resolved.[81] Older patients with significant bullous disease of the lungs can develop a pneumothorax, which may be misdiagnosed as flare of their underlying pulmonary disease. Trauma, particularly in athletes participating in contact sports, can lead to pneumothorax.[82] Other relatively common causes of secondary pneumothorax include COPD, asthma, sarcoidosis, pneumocystic pneumonia, and ARDS. Unusual causes of pneumothorax include patients with Marfan's syndrom, homocystinuria, and catamenial pneumothorax (caused by thoracic endometriosis in menstruating women).[83,84] The disorder is usually diagnosed with a combination of physical examination and CXR, but can be difficult in the patient with an abnormal baseline study. Early or small pneumothoraces may be missed as approximately 500 mL of air is needed for the lesion to be seen on plain films.[85] Ultrasound or CT scan may be confirmatory in selected cases. In severe cases of tension pneumothorax, the mediastinum can be considerably shifted away from the side with the pneumothorax.

Air can also accumulate in the mediastinum (pneumomediastinum). This diagnosis should be considered in any patient who has had instrumentation of the thoracic structures (upper endoscopy, bronchoscopy, NG tube placement, etc), but can also appear spontaneously in patients with asthma, severe cough or vomiting, and after childbirth.[86,87] Common presenting signs and symptoms include chest pain, dyspnea, and subcutaneous emphysema. Air can track a considerable distance and we have seen pneumomediastinum occur after intra-abdominal procedures like colonoscopy. Diagnosis is best confirmed with CXR and, if the diagnosis remains in doubt, cross-sectional imaging.

Pleural Effusion and Pleuritis

Patients with routine pleural effusions usually present with shortness of breath, but may have a component of chest pain, which usually but not always varies with respiration (plerutic pain). Pain is more commonly present when the effusion is inflamed, particularly if it is infected or if another exudative process such as malignancy is present.[88] Like pneumothoraces, CXR is usually diagnostic, but small effusions (both symptomatic and asymptomatic) can be missed. The etiology of pleural effusions is best ascertained by analysis of fluid obtained by thoracentesis. Patients with systemic lupus erythematosis can have pain related to inflammation of the pleura with or without a significant effusion.[89] Mesothelioma and other pleural-based malignancies may also present with chest pain.[90]

Miscellaneous

Aortic Dissection and Aneurysm

Acute aortic dissection (AD) is a medical emergency that requires prompt diagnosis and treatment.[91] If diagnosed early and correctly a survival rate of up to 75% may be expected but can be as low as 10% if left untreated.[92,93] The pain with AD usually starts suddenly and is most commonly very severe from the beginning of the pain, which is different from the crescendo pattern of cardiac pain. Most patients will have a significant history of atherosclerotic disease, but AD has been documented after athletic activity including weightlifting.[94] Plain CXR will often demonstrate an abnormal mediastinal contour suggesting the diagnosis,[95] but CT scan is the best diagnostic method with a sensitivity and specificity of close to 100%.[96] Aortic aneurysm (AA) occurs most frequently in men between 50 and 70 years of age and may involve the ascending aorta (50%), aortic arch (10%), or descending aorta (40%).[97] Most of these are asymptomatic and the development of acute chest pain suggests impending rupture and should be taken very seriously. Like AD, cross-sectional imaging using CT or MRI is the diagnostic modality of choice. If an AA becomes infected, it is said to be a mycotic aneurysm.[98] These lesions may produce pain and can be infected with several different species of bacteria and fungi. Patients present with nonspecific symptoms, often including fever and chills. A mycotic aneurysm can be seen with cross-sectional imaging, blood cultures should almost always be positive, and the organisms can occasionally be seen in a smear of the white blood cell buffy coat.

Pericarditis and Myocarditis

Pericarditis is inflammation of the fibrous sac, which surrounds the heart. The diagnosis is suggested by the combination of chest pain, a pericardial rub on examination, and typical ECG changes.[99] Pericarditis frequently follows a nonspecific viral illness, but has been associated with other, specific infectious etiologies including histoplasmosis.[100] Patients with known neoplasia, collagen vascular disease (particularly lupus), or thyroid disease have an increased incidence of this disorder.[101] Pericarditis occurs after 7 to 16% of myocardial infarctions.[102] Pain is usually sharp and sometimes varies with respiration. Relief of pain with sitting up or leaning forward is characteristic. Laboratory disorders are nonspecific, but can include leukocytosis, elevated CRP, and ESR.[103] A CXR may suggest the diagnosis, but echocardiography is confirmatory and can help guide therapy. Myocarditis can mimic acute myocardial infarction with chest pain, electrocardiographic (ECG) abnormalities, serum creatine kinase elevation, and hemodynamic instability.[104]

Pulmonary Hypertension

Pulmonary hypertension is usually caused by chronic lung disease such as COPD, although patients may present with primary disease.[105] These patients may have coexistent coronary artery disease, but some will have pain due to the right ventricular hypertrophy associated with the illness. Pain severe enough to require a nerve block for control has been reported.[106]

Herpes Zoster

The pain of herpes zoster may occur before, during, or after an outbreak of vesicular lesions. This pain is dermatomal and involves a thoracic nerve in up to 50% of cases.[107] The diagnosis is best made by history and examinations, but some patients will develop pain before their dermatologic lesions adding to the diagnostic difficulty. This pain may resolve spontaneously, but some cases will persist and require treatment with a nerve block.[108]

Drug-Induced Chest Pain

The possibility of illicit drug use should be considered in any young patient presenting with chest pain. The classic drug associated with chest pain is cocaine, which has been implicated in more than 10% of chest pain patients presenting to some emergency units.[109] Some of these patients will have demonstrable cardiac disease and even infarction, but many will have a negative cardiac evaluation. As there are often other autonomic symptoms associated with cocaine use, the patient may be wrongly diagnosed with panic disorder. Cocaine usually produces acute pain, but patients have presented with more of a chronic course.[110] Chest pain can occur after ecstasy use, perhaps due to coronary artery spasm.[111] Although technically an esophageal problem, pain from drug-induced esophagitis should be considered, particularly in patients taking tetracyclines or bisphosphonates.[112] Withdrawal symptoms can produce pain in several areas including the chest. Classically this occurs after opiate use, but has also been seen after stopping medications such as gabapentin.[113] Nitrofurantoin can produce pulmonary toxicity that is usually characterized by cough and dyspnea, but has also been associated with chest discomfort.[114]

Acute Chest Syndrome in Sickle Cell Disease

Patients with sickle cell disease (SCD) can develop a chest syndrome during a crisis characterized by severe pleuritic chest. This is felt to be caused by intracellular sickling resulting in microthromboemboli in the pulmonary circulation.[115] Pulmonary infiltrates, fever, pain, and hypoxemia are the most common symptoms, making this difficult to distinguish from pneumonia in some cases. Chest pain in patients with SCD can certainly be caused by other disorders including cardiac disease, so one should not automatically assume the etiology to be sickle cell disease.[116]

Psychological Disorders

Psychological disorders and stress can predispose to chest pain due to what is felt to be a problem with visceral hypersensitivity of the esophagus, heart, or both[117] (covered extensively in Chapter 6). Various studies suggest that 30 to 70% of noncardiac chest pain patients meet diagnostic criteria for a psychological diagnosis.[118] Some have been critical of this association on the assumption that long-term pain can produce psychological disturbances rather than the psychological problem causing the pain. In fact, depression is common even in patients with coronary disease and is also associated with increased mortality in those patients.[119] Pain in general and psychologically based chest pain in particular seem to be more common problems in women.[120] Interestingly, African-American men are more likely to think chest pain is related to their gastrointestinal tract than Caucasians, which may result in a delay in the diagnosis of heart disease in that group.[121] Hyperventilation is frequently related to anxiety, may have a component of pain, and is a very common cause of chest pain in the adolescent patient.[122]

Miscellaneous Causes

There are some other nonesophageal, noncardiac etiologies for chest pain. For example, young patients can develop a syndrome know as vocal cord dysfunction (particularly during exercise) where their cords do not relax appropriately during the respiratory cycle.[123] This symptom usually responds to speech and swallowing therapy. Patients with migraine headaches seem to have more chest symptoms but no more coronary disease than those without migraines.[124] The etiology of this is not clear, but could be due to generalized allodynia and hyperalgesia in migraine patients.[125] A mass lesion of any area within the chest cavity can produce pain. Examples include lymphoma,[126] desmoid tumor,[127] bronchogenic cyst,[128] goiter,[129] thymoma,[130] and metastatic disease.[131]

Summary

Although health care providers must respect the heart as a potentially lethal cause of chest pain and the esophagus as an area with good therapeutic options (particularly with gastroesophageal reflux-induced pain), the many noncardiac, nonesophageal etiologies must be kept in mind. Musculosketelal causes are common in both young and old chest pain patients, whether seen in the emergency room or primary care setting. The provider should maintain a high index of suspicion to recognize these conditions prior to assuming that these patients suffer from a visceral source of chest pain. Disorders of any intrathoracic or intra-abdominal organ can present with chest pain and life-threatening conditions such as pulmonary embolus and aortic dissection should be sought in appropriate patients. The diagnosis of these etiologies for pain requires the recognition of associated symptoms and signs, which will lead an astute clinician in the appropriate direction.

References

1. Wong WM, Beeler J, Risner-Adler S, et al. Attitudes and referral patterns of primary care physicians when evaluating subjects with noncardiac chest pain—A national survey. *Dig Dis Sci*. 2005;50:656-661.

2. Kupershmidt M, Varma D. Radiological tests in investigation of atypical chest pain. *Aust Fam Physician*. 2006;35:282-287.

3. Klinkman MS, Stevens D, Gorenflo DW. Episodes of care for chest pain: a preliminary report from MIRNET. *J Fam Pract*. 1994;38:345-352.

4. Buntinx F, Knockaert D, Bruyninckx R, et al. Chest pain in general practice or in the hospital emergency department: is it the same? *Fam Pract*. 2001;18:586-589.

5. Wise CM. Chest wall syndromes. Editorial review. *Curr Opin Rheumatol*. 1994;6:197-202.

6. Husser D, Bollmann A, Kuhne C, et al. Evaluation of noncardiac chest pain: diagnostic approach, coping strategies and quality of life. *Eur J Pain*. 2006;10:51-55.

7. Travell J, Rinzler SH. Pain syndromes of the chest muscles: resemblance to effort angina and myocardial infarction, and relief by local block. *Can Med Assoc J*. 1948;59:333-338.

8. Allison RD. Pain in the chest wall simulating heart disease. *Br Med J*. 1950;332-336.

9. Karlso BW, Herlitz J, Pettersson P, et al. Patients admitted to the emergency room with symptoms indicative of acute myocardial infarction. *J Intern Med*. 1991;230:251-258.

10. Levine PR, Mascette AM. Musculoskeletal chest pain in patients with angina. A prospective study. *South Med J*. 1989;82:580-585.

11. Husser D, Bollmann A, Kuhne C, et al. Evaluation of noncardiac chest pain: diagnostic approach, coping strategies and quality of life. *Eur J Pain*. 2006;10:51-55.

12. Wise CM, Semble EL, Dalton CB. Musculoskeletal chest wall syndromes in patients with noncardiac chest pain: a study of 100 patients. *Arch Phys Med Rehab*. 1992;73:147-149.

13. Ho M, Walker S, McGarry F, et al. Chest wall tenderness is unhelpful in the diagnosis of recurrent chest pain. *Quart J Med*. 2001;94:267-270.

14. Wolfe F, Smythe HA, Yunus MB, et al. The American College of Rheumatology criteria for the classification of fibromyalgia. *Arth Rheum*. 1990;33:160-172.

15. Mukerji B, Mukerji V, Alpert M, et al. The prevalence of rheumatologic disorders in patients with chest pain and angiographically normal coronary arteries. *Angiology*. 1995;46:425-430.

16. An exploratory report of chest pain in *Primary Care*. A report from ASPN. *J Am Board Fam Pract*. 1990;3:143-150.

17. Klinkman MS, Stevens D, Gorenflo DW. Episodes of chest pain: a preliminary report from MIRNET. *J Fam Pract*. 1994;38:345-352.

18. Selbst SM, Ruddy RM, Clark BJ, et al. Pediatric chest pain: a prospective study. *Pediatrics*. 1988;82:319-323.

19. Fam AG. Approach to musculoskeletal chest wall pain. *Primary Care*. 1988;15:767-782.

20. Tietze A. Uber eine eigenartige Haufung von Fallen mit Dystrophie der Rippenknorpel. *Berliner klinische Wochenschrift*. 1921;58:829-831.

21. Aeschlimann A, Kahn MF. Tietze's syndrome: a critical review. *Clin Exp Rheumatol*. 1990;8:407-412.

22. Gill G. Epidemic of Tietze's syndrome. *Br Med J*. 1977;2:499.

23. Martino F, Ettorre GC, Macarini L, et al. Diagnostic imaging of Tietze's syndrome. Comparison of computerized tomography and ultrasonography [in Italian]. *Radiologia Medica*. 1993;86:208-212.

24. Mendelson G, Mendelson H, Horowitz SF, et al. Can (99m) technetium methylene diphosphonate bone scans objectively document costochondritis? *Chest.* 1997;111:1600-1602.

25. Thongngarm T, Lemos LB, Lawhon N, Harisdangkul V. Malignant tumor with chest wall pain mimicking Tietze's syndrome. *Clin Rheumatol.* 2001;20: 276-278.

26. Cocco R, Galieni P, Bellan C, Fioravanti A. Lymphomas presenting as Tietze's syndrome: a report of 4 clinical cases. *Annali Italiani di Medicina Interna.* 1999;14:118-123.

27. Harkonen M. Tiezte's syndrome. *Br Med J.* 1977;2:1087-1089.

28. Disla E, Rhim HR, Reddy A, et al. Costochondritis: a prospective analysis in an emergency department setting. *Arch Int Med.* 1994;154:2466-2469.

29. Mendelson TG, Mendelson H, Horowitz SF, Goldfarb CR, Zumoff B. Can (99m) technetium methylene diphosphonate bone scans objectively document costochondritis? *Chest.* 1997:111:1600-1602.

30. Freeston J, Katim Z, Lindsay K, et al. Can early diagnosis and management of costochondritis reduce acute chest pain admissions? *J Rheumatol.* 2004;31: 2269-2271.

31. Wolfe F. 50 years of rheumatic therapy: the prognosis of rheumatoid arthritis. *J Rheumatol.* 1990;22:24-32.

32. Neumann L, Buskila D. Epidemiology of fibromyalgia. *Curr Pain Headache Reports.* 2003;7:362-368.

33. Pellegrino MJ. Atypical chest pain as an initial presentation of primary fibromyalgia. *Arch Phys Med Rehab.* 1990; 71:526-528.

34. Dadabhoy D, Clauw DJ. Fibromyalgia: progress in diagnosis and treatment. *Curr Pain Headache Reports.* 2005;9: 399-404.

35. Hwang E, Barkhuizen. An update on rheumatologic mimics of fibromyalgia. *Curr Pain Headache Reports.* 2006;10: 327-332.

36. Arnold LM, Hudson JI, Hess EV, et al. Family study of fibromyalgia. *Arth Rheum.* 2004;50:944-952.

37. Clauw DJ, Chrousos GP. Chronic pain and fatigue syndromes: overlapping clinical and neuroendocrine features and potential pathogenic mechanisms. *Neuroimmunomodulation.* 1997;4:134-153.

38. Staud R, Rodriguez ME. Mechanisms of disease: pain in fibromyalgia syndrome. *Nature Clin Prac Rheumatol.* 2006;2: 90-98.

39. Maresca M, Galanti G, Castellani S, et al. Pain in mitral valve prolapse. *Pain.* 1989;36:89-92.

40. Bennett R, Nelson D. Cognitive behavioral therapy for fibromyalgia. *Nature Clin Pract Rheumatol.* 2006;2:416-424.

41. Miller AJ, Texidor TA. "Precordial catch," a neglected syndrome of precordial pain. *JAMA.* 1955;159:1364-1365.

42. Gumbiner CH. Precordial catch syndrome. *South Med J.* 2003;96:38-41.

43. Cyriax EF. On various conditions that may stimulate the referred pains of visceral disease, and consideration of these from the point of view of cause and effect. *Practitioner (Lond).* 1919;102:314-322.

44. Davies-Colley R. Slipping rib. *Br Med J.* 1922:1:432.

45. Wright J. Slipping rib syndrome. *Lancet.* 1980:2:632-634.

46. Scott EM, Scott BB. Painful rib syndrome: a review of 76 cases. *Gut.* 1993;34: 1006-1008.

47. Peterson LL, Cavanaugh DG. Two years of debilitating pain in a football spearing victim: slipping rib syndrome. *Med Sci Sports Exer.* 2003;35:1634-1637.

48. Heinz GJ, Zavala DC. Slipping rib syndrome. *JAMA.* 1977;237:794-795.

49. Ryan EL. Cervicothoracic pain due to fatigue of pectoral girdle musculature. *Med J Aust.* 1991;155:204-205.

50. Brown CW, Deffer PA, Akmankjian J, et al. The natural history of thoracic disc herniation. *Spine.* 1992;17:S97-S102.

51. Sabri MR, Ghavanini AA, Haghighat M, Imanieh MH. Chest pain in children and

adolescents: epigastric tenderness as a guide to reduce unnecessary work-up. *Pediatr Cardiol.* 2003;24:3-5.

52. Ogren M, Eriksson H, Bergqvist D, Sternby NH. Subcutaneous fat accumulation and BMI associated with risk for pulmonary embolism in patients with proximal deep vein thrombosis: a population study based on 23,796 consecutive autopsies. *J Int Med.* 2005;258:166-171.

53. Ransom P, Cornelius P. Stabbing chest pain: a case of intermittent diaphragmatic herniation. *Emerg Med J.* 2005;22:460-461.

54. Sivansankaran S, Kawamura A, Lombardi D, Nesto RW. Gastric volvulus presenting as an acute coronary syndrome. *Tex Heart Inst J.* 2006;33:266-268.

55. Tan CP, Chia CH, Leese R. Chest pain in the early postoperative period after laparoscopic adjustable gastric banding. *Anesthesia.* 2006;61:390-393.

56. Lanthaler M, Sweiss H, Weissenboeck E, et al. Mediastinal emphysema after laparoscopic gastric banding. *Surg Endosc.* 2003;17:661.

57. Landen S, Majerus B, Delugeau V. Complications of gastric banding presenting to the ED. *Am J Emerg Med.* 2005;23:368-370.

58. Strasberg SM. Cholelithiasis and acute cholecystitis. *Baillieres Clin Gastroenterol.* 1997;22:643-661.

59. Mortele KJ, Wiesner W, Intriere L, et al. A modified CT severity index for evaluating acute pancreatitis: improved correlation with patient outcome. *Am J Radiol.* 2004;183:1261-1255.

60. Nayak N, Anderson JB, Channer KS. Spontaneous subcapsular renal haemorrhage presenting with pleuritic chest pain. *Urol International.* 1999;62:217-219.

61. Ek EW, Chin SL, Sutherland A, et al. Atypical chest pain and shortness of breath: rupture of an aneurysm of the left gastric artery. *ANZ J Surg.* 2005;75:834-835.

62. Knockaert DC, Buntinx F, Stoens N, et al. Chest pain in the emergency department: the broad spectrum of causes. *Eur J Emerg Med.* 2002;9;25-30.

63. Mandell LA. Epidemiology and etiology of community-acquired pneumonia. *Infect Dis Clin North Am.* 2004;18:761-776.

64. Marrie TJ. Community-acquired pneumonia. *Clin Infect Dis.* 1994;18:501-513.

65. Ponka A, Sarna S. Differential diagnosis of viral, mycoplasma and bacteraemic pneumococcal pneumonias on admission to hospital. *Eur J Respir Dis.* 1983;64(5):360-368.

66. Marais BJ, Gie RP, Obihara CC, Hesseling AC, Schaaf HS, Beyers N. Well-defined symptoms are of value in the diagnosis of childhood pulmonary tuberculosis. *Arch Dis Childhood.* 2005;90:1162-1165.

67. Kapotsis GE, Daniil Z, Malagari K, et al. A young male with chest pain, cough and fever. *Eur Resp J.* 2004;24:506-509.

68. Oymak FS, Demirbas HM, Mavili E, et al. Bronchiolitis obliterans organizing pneumonia. Clinical and roentgenological features in 26 cases. *Respiration.* 2005;72:254-262.

69. Laack TA, Goyal DG. Pulmonary embolism: an unsuspected killer. *Emerg Med Clin North Am.* 2004;22:961-983.

70. Miniati M, Prediletto R, Formichji B, et al. Accuracy of clinical assessment in the diagnosis of pulmonary embolism. *Am J Respir Crit Care Med.* 1999;159:864-871.

71. Fruergaard P, Launbjerg J, Hesse B, et al. The diagnosis of patients admitted with acute chest pain but without myocardial infarction. *Eur Heart J.* 1996;17:1028-1034.

72. Karlson BW, Herlitz J, Pettersson P, et al. Patients admitted to the emergency room with symptoms indicative of acute myocardial infarction. *J Int Med.* 1991;230:251-258.

73. Morgenthaler TI, Ryu JH. Clinical characteristics of fatal pulmonary embolism in a referral hospital. *Mayo Clin Proc.* 1995;70:417-424.

74. Laack TA, Goyal DG. Pulmonary embolism: an unsuspected killer. *Emerg Med Clin North Am*. 2004;22:961–983.

75. Dunmire SM. Pulmonary embolism. *Emerg Med Clin North Am*. 1989;7:339–354.

76. Stein PD, Hull RD, Patel K, et al. D-dimer for the exclusion of acute venous thrombosis and pulmonary embolism: a systematic review. *Ann Intern Med*. 2004;140:589–602.

77. Sadosty AT, Boie ET, Stead LG. Pulmonary embolism. *Emerg Med Clin North Am*. 2003;21:363–384.

78. Sonett JR. Local complications of non-small-cell lung cancer. *Curr Treat Options Oncol*. 2002;3:59–65.

79. Baughman RP, Lower EE, du Bois RM. Sarcoidosis. *Lancet*. 2003;361:1111–1118.

80. Lesur O, Delorme N, Fromaget JM, et al. Computed tomography in the etiologic assessment of idiopathic spontaneous pneumothorax. *Chest*. 1990;98:341–347.

81. DeVries WC, Wolfe WG. The management of spontaneous pneumothorax and bullous emphysema. *Surg Clin North Am*. 1989;66:851–866.

82. Perron AD. Chest pain in athletes. *Clin Sports Med*. 2003;22:37–50.

83. Yellin A, Shiner RJ, Lieberman Y. Familial multiple bilateral pneumothorax associated with Marfan syndrome. *Chest*. 1991;100(2):577–578.

84. Alifano M, Roth T, Broet SC, et al. Catamenial pneumothorax: a prospective study. *Chest*. 2003; 124(3):781–782.

85. Carr JJ, Reed JC, Choplin RH, et al. Plain and computed radiography for detecting experimentally induced pneumothorax in cadavers: implications for detection in patients. *Radiology*. 1992;183:193–199.

86. Panacek EA, Singer AJ, Sherman BW, et al. Spontaneous pneumomediastinum: clinical and natural history. *Ann Emerg Med*. 1992;21:1222–1227.

87. Butler KH, Swencki SA. Chest pain: a clinical assessment. *Radiol Clin North Am*. 2006;44:165–179.

88. Chapman SJ, Davies RJ. Pleural effusions. *Clin Med*. 2004;4:207–210.

89. Ben-Horin S, Portnoy O, Pauzner R, Livneh A. Localized pericardial inflammation in systemic lupus erythematosus. *Clin Exper Rheumatol*. 2004;22:483–484.

90. Ameille J, Matrat M, Paris C, et al. Asbestos-related pleural diseases: dimensional criteria are not appropriate to differentiate diffuse pleural thickening from pleural plaques. *Am J Indust Med*. 2004;45:289–296.

91. Pretre R, von Segesser LK. Aortic dissection. *Lancet*. 1997;349:1461–1464.

92. Jeudy J, Waite S, White CS. Nontraumatic thoracic emergencies. *Radiol Clin North Am*. 2006;44:273–293.

93. Rigolin YH, Harrison JK, Wilson JS, Bashore T. Update on aortic dissection. *Emerg Med*. 1993;18:17–35.

94. Ragucci MV, Thistle HG. Weight lifting and type II aortic dissection. A case report. *J Sports Med Physic Fitness*. 2004;44:424–427.

95. Hagan PG, Nienaber CA, Isselbacher EM, et al. The International Registry of Acute Aortic Dissection (IRAD): new insights into an old disease. *JAMA*. 2000;283:897–903.

96. Knaut AL, Cleveland Jr JC. Aortic emergencies. *Emerg Med Clin North Am*. 2003;21:817–845.

97. Bickerstaff LK, Pairolero PC, Hollier LH, et al. Thoracic aortic aneurysms: a population based study. *Surgery*. 1982;92:1103–1108.

98. Long R, Guzman R, Greenberg H, et al. Tuberculous mycotic aneurysm of the aorta: review of published medical and surgical experience. *Chest*. 1999;115:522–531.

99. Troughton RW, Asher CR, Klein AL. Pericarditis. *Lancet*. 2004;363:717–727.

100. Wang JJ. Reimold SC. Chest pain resulting from histoplasmosis pericarditis: a brief report and review of the literature. *Cardiol Review*. 2006;14:223–226.

101. Levy PY, Maotti JP, Gauduchon V, et al. Comparison of intuitive versus system-

atic strategies for aetiological diagnosis of pericardial effusion. *Scand J Infect Dis.* 2005;37:216-220.

102. Shabetai R. Acute pericarditis. *Cardiol Clin.* 1990;8:639-644.

103. Lange RA, Hillis LD. Acute pericarditis. *N Engl J Med.* 2004;351:2195-2202.

104. Dec GW Jr, Waldman H, Southern J, et al. Viral myocarditis mimicking acute myocardial infarction. *J Am Coll Cardiol.* 1992;20:85-89.

105. Rubin LJ. Pathology and pathophysiology of primary pulmonary hypertension. *Am J Cardiol.* 1995;7(suppl 5):51A-54A.

106. Parris WC, Lin S, Frist W Jr. Use of stellate ganglion blocks for chronic chest pain associated with primary pulmonary hypertension. *Anesth Analg.* 1988;67:993-995.

107. Wise CM, Semble EL, Dalton CB. Musculoskeletal chest wall syndromes in patients with noncardiac chest pain: a study of 100 patients. *Arch Phys Med Rehab.* 1992;73:147-149.

108. Doi K, Nikai T, Sakura S, Saito Y. Intercostal nerve block with 5% tetracaine for chronic pain syndromes. *J Clin Anesthesia.* 2002;14:39-41.

109. Hollander JE, Todd KH, Green G, et al. Chest pain associated with cocaine: an assessment of prevalence in suburban and urban emergency departments. *Ann Emerg Med.* 1995;26:671-676.

110. Jones JH, Weir WB. Cocaine-induced chest pain. *Clin Lab Med.* 2006;26:127-146.

111. Bassi S. Rittoo D. Ecstacy and chest pain due to coronary artery spasm. *Inter J Cardiol.* 2005;99:485-487.

112. Kadayifci A, Gulsen MT, Koruk M, Savas MC. Doxycycline-induced pill esophagitis. *Dis Esoph.* 2004;17:168-171.

113. Tran KT, Hranicky D, Lark T, Jacob NJ. Gabapentin withdrawal syndrome in the presence of a taper. *Bipolar Dis.* 2005;7:302-304.

114. Liesching T, O'Brien A. Dyspnea, chest pain, and cough: the lurking culprit. Nitrofurantoin-induced pulmonary toxicity. *Postgrad Med.* 2002;112:19-20.

115. Castro O, Brambilla DJ, Thorington B, et al. The acute chest syndrome in sickle cell disease: incidence and risk factors. *Blood.* 1994;84:643-649.

116. Haynes J, Kirkpatrick MB. The acute chest syndrome of sickle cell disease. *Am J Med Sci.* 1993;305:326-329.

117. Carter CS, Servan-Schreiber D, Perlstein WM. Anxiety disorders and the syndrome of chest pain with normal coronary arteries: prevalence and pathophysiology. *Clin Psychiatry.* 1997;58:S70-S73.

118. Katon W, Hall ML, Russo J, Hollifield M, Vitaliano PP, Beitman BD. Chest pain: relationship of psychiatric illness to coronary arteriographic results. *Am Med.* 1988;84:1-9.

119. Frasure-Smith N, Lesperance F, Talajic M. Depression and 18-month prognosis after myocardial infarction. *Circulation.* 1995;91:999-1005.

120. Sheps DS, Creed F, Clouse RE. Chest pain in patients with cardiac and noncardiac disease. *Psychosomatic Med.* 2004;66:861-867.

121. Klingler D, Green-Weir R, Nerenz D, et al. Perceptions of chest pain differ by race. *Am Heart J.* 2002;144:51-59.

122. Pantell RH, Goodman BW. Adolescent chest pain: a prospective study. *Pediatrics.* 1983;71:881-887.

123. Truwit J. Pulmonary disorders and exercise. *Clin Sports Med.* 2003;22:161-180.

124. Logroscino G, Lipton RB. Migraine is associated with chest symptoms but not cardiac events. A reassuring paradox. *Neurology.* 2004;63:2209-2210.

125. Sarkar S, Aziz Q, Woolf CJ, et al. Contribution of central sensitization to the development of non-cardiac chest pain. *Lancet.* 2000;356:1154-1159.

126. Premkumar V, Paimany B, Gopal AS. Primary large B-cell cardiac lymphoma. *J Am Soc Echocardio.* 2006;19:107.

127. de Jong WK, van der Graaf WT, van der Jagt EJ, et al. A 20-year-old male with thoracic pain and a lower thoracic mass. Diagnosis: intrathoracal desmoid tumour with microscopically incomplete resection. *Eur Respir J*. 2005;26: 740-743.

128. Georghiou GP, Vidne BA, Saute M. Bronchogenic cyst: an unusual cause of acute retrosternal pain. *Asian Cardiovasc Thorac Ann*. 2005;13:99.

129. Iacobellis G. Huge mediastinal goiter: an unusual cause of precordial pain. *Thyroid*. 2004;14:635.

130. Santana L, Givica A, Camacho C. Armed Forces Institute of Pathology. Best cases from the AFIP: thymoma. *Radiographics*. 2002;22:S95-S102.

131. Yasuda N, Ishiki R, Agetsuma H. Single large metastatic tumor growing progressively and occupying right ventricular cavity. *Heart*. 2002;87:328.

CHAPTER 5

Sensory Testing in Noncardiac Chest Pain

Abhishek Sharma
Qasim Aziz

Background

Patients with noncardiac chest pain (NCCP) represent a complex and heterogeneous group. In these patients, in whom a cardiac cause for pain is believed to have been excluded, the esophagus is the most common source of symptoms with the majority (up to 60%) having evidence of gastroesophageal reflux disease (GERD) and a smaller proportion demonstrating esophageal dysmotility.[1] The remainder often demonstrate a heightened sensitivity to experimental esophageal stimulation, termed visceral hypersensitivity (VH). This heightened sensitivity, which manifests as lowered perceptual and/or pain thresholds to a variety of intraesophageal stimuli, is believed to be important in the generation and maintenance of symptoms in this disorder; however, the mechanisms that underlie it remain unclear.

Although treatments exist for reflux disease and esophageal dysmotility, therapeutic options for those with visceral hypersensitivity remain limited. Accurately profiling the sensory dysfunction in these patients to better understand the mechanisms involved in pain transduction, transmission, and perception and the activities of distinct visceral afferent nociceptive pathways is a crucial step along the journey to novel drug discovery. This, in turn, is sorely needed given the considerable burden of disease posed by NCCP.

The Modalities for Sensory Testing in the Esophagus

The process leading to the conscious perception of intraesophageal stimuli begins with the activation of visceral afferent fibers and their receptors. The receptors on esophageal afferent fibers have been classified both on their location within the layers of the viscera into mucosal receptors and muscle receptors, and on the basis of the sensory modality they are responsive to into mechano-, chemo-, and thermoreceptors.[2] Studies in humans have shown that the esophagus can sense mechanical, electrical, chemical, and thermal stimuli, and some of these sensory modalities have been applied to qualify sensory dysfunctions in patients with NCCP. The experience with each sensory modality is considered in turn.

Esophageal Distension

The esophagus distends in response to food and often with gastroesophageal reflux, and this can produce a variety of symptoms including heartburn and chest pain. It is therefore not surprising that mechanical distension of the viscera with a balloon or a barostat represents one of the most extensively studied modalities of sensory testing. In fact, Hertz in 1911 was the first to report that balloon distension in the esophagus could induce chest pain.[3] It was later documented that esophageal balloon distension in patients with ischemic heart disease reproduced anginal pain, but without ischemic electrocardiographic changes.[4] Low levels of distension in the esophagus often induce secondary peristalsis whereas higher levels induce symptoms via activation of mechanosensitive afferents in vagal and spinal nerves.[5]

Studies in the opossum esophagus by Sengupta et al have demonstrated two types of low-threshold vagal afferent fibers. The first type exhibit short-duration activity in response to swallows which correlates with contractions of the circular muscle layer, whereas the second type show a long duration of response during swallows which correlates with longitudinal muscle contractions.[6] Vagal afferent fibers exhibit a steep increase in their activity within a narrow range of distending pressure, implying that they are responsible for physiologic processes and reflexes within the esophagus.[7] In contrast, spinal afferents contain both low- and high-threshold mechanosensitive fibers that demonstrate a linear increase in activity to increasing levels of distension.[5,7] It has been proposed that the pain evoked by esophageal distension is mediated by spinal afferents through the recruitment of high-threshold mechanonociceptors.[5]

The seminal study of intraesophageal balloon distension in patients with NCCP was performed by Richter et al in 1986.[8] In 30 patients and 30 controls they progressively inflated a balloon in the distal esophagus at 1-mL intervals, and found that 60% of patients reported chest pain compared with 20% of controls ($p < 0.005$). In addition, 50% of patients reported pain at balloon volumes of 8 mL or less, whereas controls only reported pain at volumes of 9 mL or more, suggesting the presence of visceral hypersensitivity in these patients (Fig 5–1). There were no differences in esophageal contractility, tone, or balloon pressures between groups.

The above findings were reproduced by Rao et al who studied patients with NCCP using impedance planimetry, a technique that allows simultaneous measurement of esophageal cross-sectional area (CSA) and intraluminal pressure, and facilitates calculation of some of the biomechanical properties of the esophageal wall.[9] In 24 NCCP patients and 12 healthy controls, stepwise balloon dis-

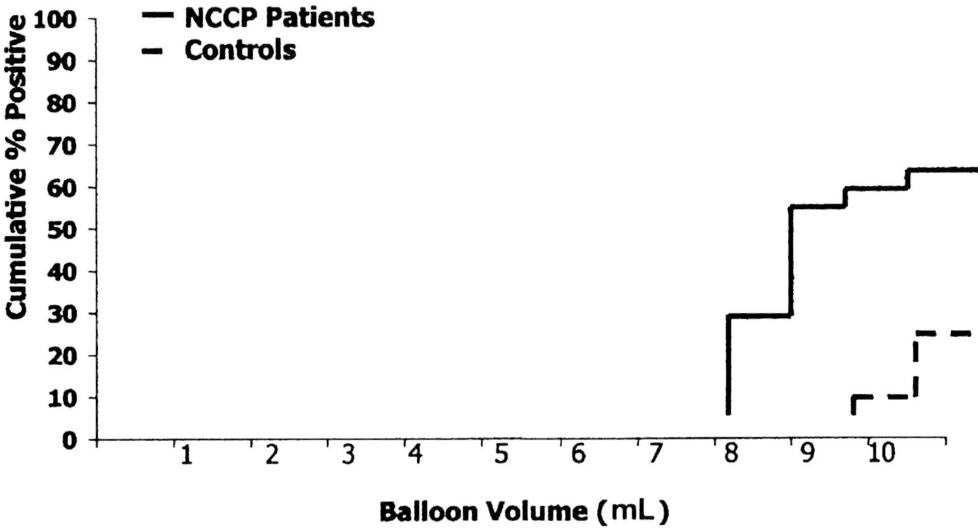

Fig 5–1. Visceral hypersensitivity in NCCP. Patients with NCCP report pain at lower volumes of distal esophageal balloon distension compared to normal controls. (Reprinted from *Gastroenterology*, Volume 91 (4), Richter JE, Barish CF, Castell DO. Abnormal sensory perception in patients with esophageal chest pain. Pages 845–852. Copyright 1986, with permissiion from the American Gastroenterological Association.

tension induced first sensation at significantly lower pressures in patients compared to controls (p <0.001). Moderate discomfort and typical chest pain were reported in 83% of patients but by none of the controls (p <0.001). Although they also reported that the esophageal wall was less distensible (compliant) compared to controls, they subsequently demonstrated the persistence of hypersensitivity to intraesophageal balloon distension and the tendency to develop chest pain despite relaxation of the muscle wall with atropine.[9,10]

Some light has been shed on the mechanism of pain to intraesophageal balloon distension in NCCP by de Caestecker et al.[11] They performed 1-mL stepwise balloon distensions in 13 patients with NCCP with esophageal motility disorders and 10 healthy volunteers before and after the administration of intravenous edrophonium and atropine. Although there were no differences between the groups in the distending volume at perception of discomfort, edrophonium resulted in a significant reduction in distension threshold for pain in patients. In both controls and patients, the distension volume for pain after atropine was significantly higher than after edrophonium. It was therefore proposed that the pain receptor for noxious stretch and after edrophonium challenge was an "in series" mechanoreceptor located in esophageal longitudinal muscle.[11]

Although the studies above have highlighted some of the experience with intraesophageal balloon distension it is important to add that distension by gas also has been postulated as a cause for pain in some NCCP patients. Gignoux et al performed intraesophageal balloon distensions and a study of the belching reflex provoked by intraesophageal air injection in 54 patients and 33 controls.[12]

They were then stratified into high-threshold (group 1) and low-threshold (group 2) belchers depending on if they belched during two of three 40-mL distensions or not. Balloon distension induced pain in 64% of the patients in group I, and in 14% of the patients in group 2 ($p < 0.01$). High-threshold belching seemed to be a factor favoring the likelihood of experiencing pain on intraesophageal balloon distension. They postulated that esophageal distension by air due to a belching disorder might be the mechanism responsible for pain in some NCCP patients with heightened sensitivity to balloon distension.[12]

Electrical Stimulation

Depolarization of afferent fibers by electrical current has been widely used as an experimental stimulus throughout the gut and has proven to be safe, reliable, and reproducible.[13-15] Electrical stimulators connected to specially designed stimulation catheters with mucosal contact points can deliver varying intensities of electrical current at different frequencies, waveforms, and durations evoking different kinds of pain.[16] In addition, the well-defined onset and offset of the stimulus ensures a short latency to afferent fiber stimulation and is useful for temporal correlations. It is this latter property that makes it attractive in the assessment of cortical evoked potentials which are discussed later.

Another advantage of electrical stimulation is the ability to easily assess temporal summation or "wind-up," which is a progressive, frequency-dependent facilitation of neuronal responses in response to repetitive stimuli of constant intensity often causing an increasing perception of pain.[17] In the majority of the literature wind-up has been induced by electrical stimulation.[17] Wind-up is a useful research tool as it shares some of the same mechanisms and receptor processes as central sensitization, being attenuated by N-methyl-D-aspartate (NMDA) receptor antagonists.[18] A potential disadvantage of electrical stimulation is that it bypasses the receptors and depolarizes all afferent nerve fibers directly, and hence cannot be used to infer activity in specific nociceptors.

Most studies assessing esophageal electrical pain thresholds in NCCP have been performed before and after chemical exposure (most often with acid) to assess the characteristics of sensitization, which is now discussed.

Chemical Stimulation

Chemical stimulation of the gastrointestinal (GI) tract, like mechanical distension, represents potentially a "physiologic stimulus" with the added advantage of being able to induce mucosal changes akin to inflammation. In the esophagus the most utilized irritant has been acid, although other substances have been used in other parts of the GI tract including, glycerol,[19] capsaicin,[20] and hypertonic saline.[21] Esophageal acid infusion can produce symptoms of heartburn, discomfort, and chest pain,[22] and for some time was used as a diagnostic test for esophagitis and NCCP.[23,24] With the advent of pH testing and later the proton-pump inhibitor test, esophageal acid perfusion is now mainly used to sensitize the esophagus to subsequent sensory testing.

Mehta et al studied 25 patients with NCCP and divided them into those with positive or negative results on esophageal provocation tests.[25] After acid perfusion, balloon perception and pain thresholds decreased in patients with negative results on esophageal tests and in controls but not in patients with positive results on esophageal tests. They hypothesised that the lack of sensitization in patients with positive results on esophageal provocation testing indicated that their esophageal nociceptors were already sensitized.[25]

Peghini et al subsequently reported in healthy volunteers that only those subjects that reported heartburn or chest pain during intraesophageal acid infusion, so termed "acid-sensitive," developed sensitization to balloon distension with a fall in pain thresholds.[26] In contrast, DeVault et al later reported in healthy volunteers that a 15-minute infusion of 0.1N HCl had no effect on pain thresholds to subsequent intraesophageal balloon distension.[27] These studies served to demonstrate the inherent variability in sensory responses after chemical sensitization with acid.

Using an alternative sensory testing modality, Sarkar et al documented a fall in electrical pain thresholds in the proximal esophagus and anterior chest wall, the somatic site of pain referral, in healthy volunteers after distal esophageal acidification. In comparison, patients with NCCP not only had lower resting esophageal pain thresholds, but also an exaggerated response to esophageal acid with their pain thresholds falling further and for longer (mean fall in area under threshold/time curve 26.7 [11.0–42.3] vs 5.8 [2.8–8.8] units; $p = 0.04$, Fig 5-2).[28] The development of hyperalgesia in both the nonacid exposed proximal esophagus and anterior chest wall following distal esophageal acidification suggests that central sensitization may contribute to visceral pain disorders. It was proposed that the prolonged hyperalgesia in patients with NCCP represented a central enhancement of nociceptive processing.[28]

With the above model, subsequent studies in healthy volunteers have demonstrated that acid-induced proximal esophageal secondary hyperalgesia can be attenuated by prostaglandin E2 receptor-1 (EP-1) receptor antagonists,[29] and both prevented and reversed with N-methyl D-aspartate (NMDA) receptor antagonism.[30] Further evaluation of these novel compounds in patients with NCCP is therefore warranted.

An important issue with chemical stimulation, such as esophageal acidification, is that there is both interindividual variation in the magnitude of hyperalgesia that develops and intraindividual variation in this response between visits.[31] In addition, with electrical sensory testing a proportion of individuals fail to sensitize to acid and around 14% habituate with diminishing sensitization to repeated acid infusions.[31] Nonsensitization to intraesophageal balloon distension postesophageal acidification has already been discussed.[27] The factors that determine the degree to which an individual develops visceral hyperalgesia in response to esophageal acidification, why some do not develop it at all, and why some habituate are not known; however, recent studies have uncovered some underlying physiologic variations that may account for phenotypic differences.

For instance, Tougas et al assessed autonomic activity using the validated technique of power spectral analysis of heart rate variability (PSHRV), before and during esophageal acidification with 0.1N HCl in 28 NCCP patients and 10 matched healthy controls. Vagal and sympathetic activity were assessed by standard

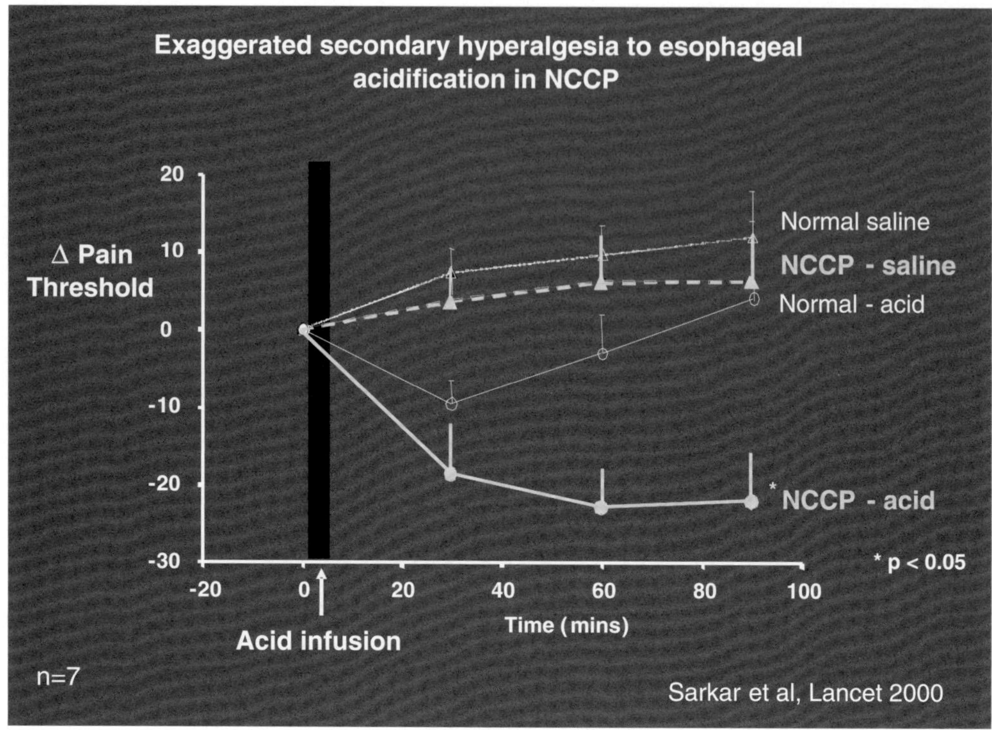

Fig 5–2. Exaggerated secondary hyperalgesia to esophageal acidification in NCCP. The above shows the mean change in pain threshold in upper esophagus of seven patients with NCCP and six healthy controls after a 5 min infusion of acid or saline into the lower esophagus. The exaggerated and prolonged sensitization shown by patients with NCCP in response to a short period of acid infusion raises the possibility that a shift in the way the central nervous system handles peripheral sensory input contributes to the pathophysiology of the chest symptoms. (Adapted from Sarkar S, Aziz Q, Woolf CJ, Hobson AR, Thompson DG. Contribution of central sensitisation to the development of non-cardiac chest pain. *Lancet*. 2000;356:1154–1159; with permission from Elsevier.)

high frequency (HF) (0.15–0.5 Hz) and low-frequency (LF) (0.06–0.15 Hz) PSHRV indices, respectively. A total of 19/28 patients had angina-like symptoms elicited by acid, and these "acid sensitive" patients had a higher baseline heart rate (82.9 [3.1 SEM] vs 66.7 [3.5 SEM] beats per min; p <0.005) and lower baseline vagal activity (p <0.03) than "acid insensitive" patients. In addition, vagal cardiac outflow increased (p <0.03) in acid sensitive but not acid insensitive patients during acid infusion. It was concluded that acid sensitive NCCP patients have

decreased resting vagal activity that increases with esophageal acidification, and that the elicited symptoms were in keeping with a vagally mediated "pseudoaffective response."[32]

Interestingly, prior to the above, Hollerbach et al reported a greater degree of reduction in sympathetic outflow and increase in cardiovagal activity on electrical esophageal stimulation (EOS) in NCCP patients compared to controls.[33] During EOS heart rate decreased in NCCP patients but not in controls (p <0.003). It was concluded that the hypersensitivity to EOS in NCCP patients was associated with a greater cardiovagal reflex response.[33]

Differences in autonomic reactivity to esophageal acidification have also been reported in both GERD and NERD patients although with conflicting results, thereby limiting the inferences that can be made on how autonomic function modulates sensory perception from the esophagus.[34,35]

Thermal Stimulation

Most individuals can differentiate thermal stimuli in the esophagus, and in some patients with esophageal pathology such as esophagitis they can induce heartburn. Drewes et al assessed sensitivity to electrical, mechanical, and thermal stimuli in the esophagus with a multimodal catheter (Fig 5-3) in 11 healthy volunteers and documented nonpainful and painful local and referred sensations to all forms of stimuli.[15] Using this multimodal assessment technique, they subsequently demonstrated allodynia to both cold and heat stimuli in the esophagus following sensitization with acid along with hyperalgesia to both electrical and mechanical stimuli.[36]

More recently, Pedersen et al documented a reduced tolerance for heat and

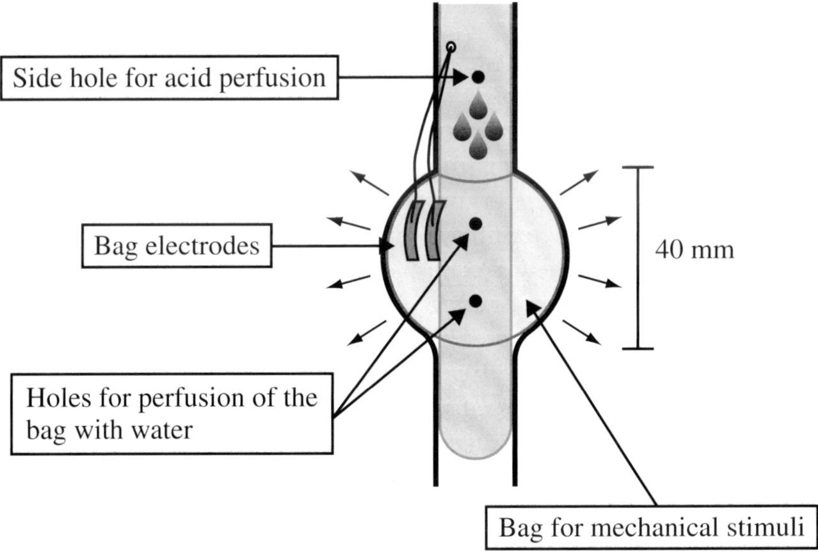

Fig 5–3. Illustration of the multimodal esophageal catheter for electrical, mechanical, heat, and cold stimuli. An inflatable bag delivers mechanical and thermal stimuli. Electrodes mounted on the outer surface of the bag deliver electrical stimuli. A 5-mm side hole proximal to the bag allows chemical stimulation, such as perfusion with acid. (Reprinted from Drewes AM, Schipper K-P, Dimcevski G, Petersen P, Andersen OK, Gregersen H, Arendt-Nielsen L. Multi-modal induction and assessment of allodynia and hyperalgesia in the human oesophagus. *Eur J. Pain*. 2003;7: 539-549. Copyright 2003, with permission from the European Federation of Chapters of the International Association for the Study of Pain.)

a greater referred pain area as opposed to cold stimuli in healthy subjects.[37] Following esophageal acidification, however, there was a fall in tolerance to heat stimuli with exaggerated referred pain areas, but no changes to cold stimuli.

To the best of our knowledge, no studies have yet assessed esophageal thermosensitivity in patients with NCCP, although one would imagine they would demonstrate hypersensitivity to this modality as well given their sensory responses to other experimental stimuli. Given the increasing interest in the transient receptor potential vanilloid type 1 (TRPV1) receptor, a nonselective cation channel expressed by sensory nerves and sensitive to heat, hydrogen ions, and capsaicin, this is likely to change.[38,39] It has already been found to be upregulated in patients with esophagitis.[40]

Evoked Potentials

Cortical evoked potentials reflect the central nervous processing of peripheral nerve activation and are routinely used in clinical practice to test visual, auditory, and somatosensory afferent pathways.[41-43] They are recorded via electrodes placed on the scalp and represent the sequence of negative (N) and positive (P) voltage changes generated in the brain following the arrival of a sensory stimulus. Latencies are described as the time in milliseconds from the stimulus onset to the first peak. Initial CEP components reflect the characteristics of the conducting afferent pathways whereas subsequent components relate to specific later steps in cortical processing.[44]

Evoked potentials have also been elicited to experimental esophageal stimuli and can be used to infer the integrity and characteristics of central nervous pathways activated by esophageal afferents. For this reason they represent a valuable addition to an investigator's armory when assessing sensory dysfunction in patients with NCCP.

Both electrical and mechanical stimuli have been used to elicit reproducible esophageal evoked potentials (EEP), although findings have been disparate even in healthy subjects. For instance, Hollerbach et al recorded reproducible evoked potentials with both modalities but documented different latencies and conduction velocities.[45] The calculated conduction velocities for both modes of stimulation (balloon: 1.73 ± 0.9 m/sec vs electrical: 10.1 ± 3.4 m/sec) were stated to be compatible with conduction through C-fibers and A-delta fibers, respectively. In contrast, Hobson et al, who also characterized EEP in response to electrical and mechanical stimulation, found that the conduction velocities (7.9-8.6 m/sec) were compatible with conduction through thinly myelinated A-delta fibers.[44] EEP amplitudes were found to be significantly smaller with mechanical as compared to electrical stimuli at the same levels of perception, implying that the latter modality activates a larger number of afferents (Fig 5-4). There was also a short latency delay with mechanical EEP compared to the counterpart electrical EEP consistent with the time delay for the former to distend the esophageal wall sufficient to trigger the afferent volley.[44]

In patients with NCCP, three studies have documented lower EEP amplitudes to electrical and balloon distension protocols.[33,46,47] In one of these, Smout et al reported lower amplitudes and longer latencies of EEP components evoked to esophageal balloon distension in patients with NCCP compared to controls; however, adjustments for the fact that smaller

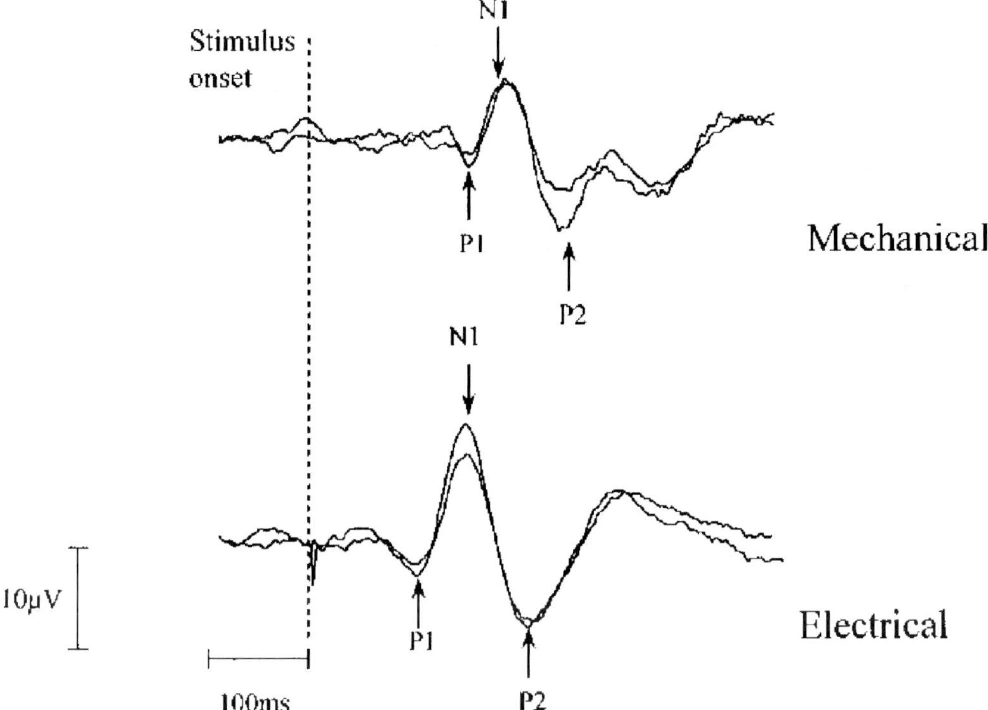

Fig 5–4. Normal cortical-evoked potential morphology. Figure shows cortical evoked potential morphology in response to mechanical and electrical stimulation in one subject. The superimposed traces represent the same study on a second occasion and demonstrate the reproducibility of each component. A similar triphasic response can be seen with both stimuli. P1 = 1st positive component; N1 = 1st negative component; P2 = 2nd positive component. (Used with permission from Hobson AR, Sarkar S, Furlong PL, Thompson DG, Aziz Q. A cortical evoked potential study of afferents mediating human esophageal sensation. *Am J Physiol Gastrointest Liver Physiol.* 2000;279: G139–G147.)

volumes of air were required to produce sensations in NCCP compared to controls revealed that the amplitude and quality of the EEP was no longer different between groups.[46] It was proposed that the heightened perception of esophageal distension in patients with NCCP was caused by altered central processing rather than abnormal or up-regulated receptors in the esophageal wall.[46]

Hollerbach et al reported shorter EEP latencies to electrical esophageal stimulation and more pronounced changes of the outflow of the autonomic nervous system (ANS) in NCCP patients.[33] Frobert et al also demonstrated shorter latencies and lower amplitudes of the somatosensory EP from the anterior chest wall in NCCP patients.[47] These findings also suggest increased central nervous system responsiveness to visceral stimuli in patients with NCCP similar to that found in other FGD patients.

Most recently, Sarkar et al demonstrated it was possible to potentiate EEP components after esophageal injury. They reported an increase in sensitivity of the proximal esophageal afferent pathway following distal esophageal acidification associated with a reduction in the latency of the EEP response.[48] This provided objective, neurophysiologic evidence of the role of central sensitization in their model of acid-induced visceral pain hypersensitivity (Fig 5–5).

Hobson and Aziz have suggested that different subgroups of patients with NCCP may exist, namely, those with short latency early EEP components having sensitization of gastrointestinal afferent pathways, and those with long latencies and enhanced late responses with hypervigilance and increased affective processing.[49] Subsequently, they were able to subclassify NCCP patients into distinct phenotypes based on sensory responsiveness and EEP morphology.[50] NCCP patients with esophageal hypersensitivity were subdivided into those with normal/reduced latencies (group 1) and those with increased latencies (group 2). A third group had normal pain thresholds with normal or increased P1 latencies. It was proposed that patients with

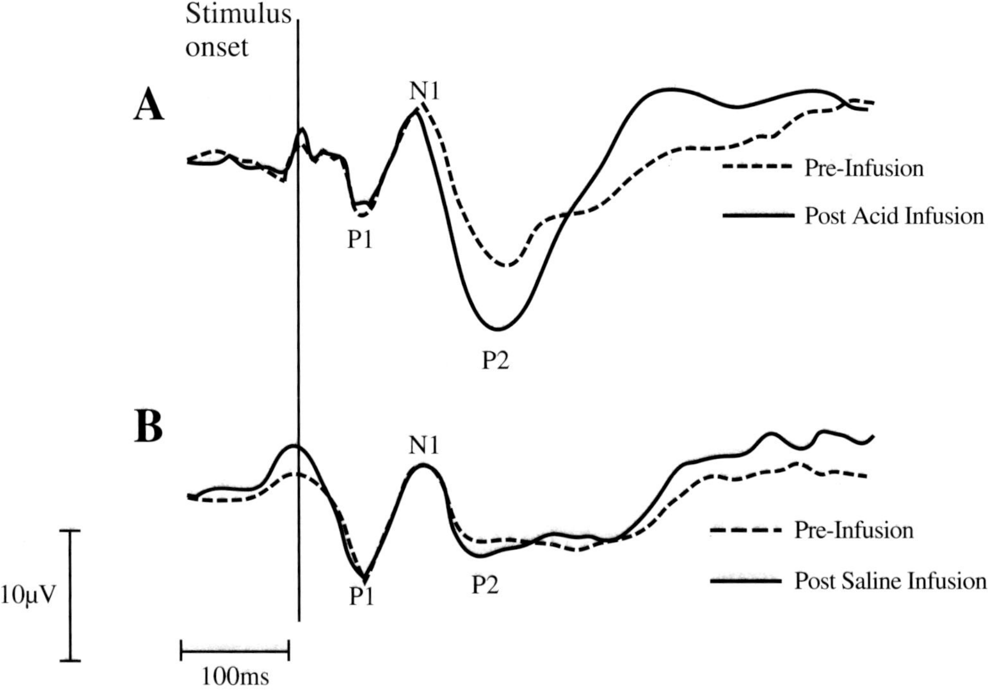

Fig 5–5. Increased proximal esophageal afferent pathway sensitivity following distal esophageal acidification. Distal esophageal acid infusion is associated with a reduction in latency of the EEP response from the nonacid exposed proximal esophagus. No change in latency occurs following saline infusion. These results support the involvement of central sensitization in the mediation of visceral pain hypersensitivity. (Reproduced with permission from Sarkar S, Hobson AR, Furlong PL, et al. Central neural mechanisms mediating human visceral hypersensitivity. *Am J Physiol Gastrointest Liver Physiol.* 2001;281(5):G1196–G1202.)

the group 1 phenotype had enhanced esophageal afferent pathway sensitivity whereas those with the group 2 phenotype had normal afferent transmission to the cortex but subsequent heightened secondary cortical processing of this information compatible with psychological factors such as hypervigilance.[50]

Summary and Future Directions

As one can see from the above, in the last 20 years major developments have been made in the sensory evaluation of patients with NCCP. A range of modalities are now available at the hands of the investigator to characterize the sensory dysfunction in these patients, such as intraesophageal balloon distension, and electrical and thermal stimulation. These in turn may be combined with cortical evoked potentials to further characterize afferent pathway sensitivity.

Our early experience with these modalities has already served to highlight the variability in both health and disease. It seems unlikely that NCCP is a homogeneous disorder, and more likely that it is composed of different pathophysiologic phenotypes, with varying degrees of visceral hypersensitivity, psychological comorbidity, and possibly autonomic dysfunction. At present we must focus on characterizing these phenotypes with multimodal sensory evaluation, study of psychological and autonomic profiles, and documentation of evoked potential morphology. These efforts, incorporated with other future developments, will ensure patients receive the most appropriate and targeted therapeutic options.

References

1. Richter JE, Bradley LA, Castell DO. Esophageal chest pain: current controversies in pathogenesis, diagnosis, and therapy. *Ann Intern Med.* 1989;110(1): 66-78.
2. Gebhart GF. Pathobiology of visceral pain: molecular mechanisms and therapeutic implications IV. Visceral afferent contributions to the pathobiology of visceral pain. *Am J Physiol Gastrointest Liver Physiol.* 2000;278(6):G834-G838.
3. Hertz A. The sensibility of the alimentary tract in health and disease. *Lancet.* 1911; 1:1051-1056.
4. Lipkin M SM. Studies of visceral pain: measurements of stimulus intensity and duration associated with the onset of pain in esophagus, ileum and colon. *J Clin Invest.* 1957;37:28-34.
5. Sengupta JN. An overview of esophageal sensory receptors. *Am J Med.* 2000; 108(suppl 4a):87S-89S.
6. Sengupta JN, Kauvar D, Goyal RK. Characteristics of vagal esophageal tension-sensitive afferent fibers in the opossum. *J Neurophysiol.* 1989;61(5):1001-1010.
7. Sengupta JN, Saha JK, Goyal RK. Stimulus-response function studies of esophageal mechanosensitive nociceptors in sympathetic afferents of opossum. *J Neurophysiol.* 1990;64(3):796-812.
8. Richter JE, Barish CF, Castell DO. Abnormal sensory perception in patients with esophageal chest pain. *Gastroenterology.* 1986;91(4):845-852.
9. Rao SS, Gregersen H, Hayek B, Summers RW, Christensen J. Unexplained chest pain: the hypersensitive, hyperreactive, and poorly compliant esophagus. *Ann Intern Med.* 1996;124(11):950-958.
10. Rao SS, Hayek B, Summers RW. Functional chest pain of esophageal origin: hyperalgesia or motor dysfunction. *Am J Gastroenterol.* 2001;96(9):2584-2589.
11. de Caestecker JS, Pryde A, Heading RC. Site and mechanism of pain perception

with oesophageal balloon distension and intravenous edrophonium in patients with oesophageal chest pain. *Gut.* 1992; 33(5):580–586.

12. Gignoux C, Bost R, Hostein J, et al. Role of upper esophageal reflex and belch reflex dysfunctions in noncardiac chest pain. *Dig Dis Sci.* 1993;38(10):1909–1914.

13. Accarino AM, Azpiroz F, Malagelada JR. Symptomatic responses to stimulation of sensory pathways in the jejunum. *Am J Physiol.* 1992;263(5 pt 1):G673–G677.

14. Drewes AM, Petersen P, Qvist P, Nielsen J, Arendt-Nielsen L. An experimental pain model based on electric stimulations of the colon mucosa. *Scand J Gastroenterol.* 1999;34(8):765–771.

15. Drewes AM, Schipper KP, Dimcevski G, et al. Multimodal assessment of pain in the esophagus: a new experimental model. *Am J Physiol Gastrointest Liver Physiol.* 2002;283(1):G95–G103.

16. Le Bars D, Gozariu M, Cadden SW. Animal models of nociception. *Pharmacol Rev.* 2001;53(4):597–652.

17. Herrero JF, Laird JM, Lopez-Garcia JA. Wind-up of spinal cord neurones and pain sensation: much ado about something? *Prog Neurobiol.* 2000;61(2):169–203.

18. Woolf CJ, Thompson SW. The induction and maintenance of central sensitization is dependent on N-methyl-D-aspartic acid receptor activation; implications for the treatment of post-injury pain hypersensitivity states. *Pain.* 1991;44(3):293–299.

19. Bouin M, Delvaux M, Blanc C, et al. Intrarectal injection of glycerol induces hypersensitivity to rectal distension in healthy subjects without modifying rectal compliance. *Eur J Gastroenterol Hepatol.* 2001;13(5):573–580.

20. Drewes AM, Schipper KP, Dimcevski G, et al. Gut pain and hyperalgesia induced by capsaicin: a human experimental model. *Pain.* 2003;104(1–2):333–341.

21. Drewes AM, Babenko L, Birket-Smith L, Funch-Jensen P, Arendt-Nielsen L. Induction of non-painful and painful intestinal sensations by hypertonic saline: a new human experimental model. *Eur J Pain.* 2003;7(1):81–91.

22. Howard PJ, Maher L, Pryde A, Heading RC. Symptomatic gastro-oesophageal reflux, abnormal oesophageal acid exposure, and mucosal acid sensitivity are three separate, though related, aspects of gastro-oesophageal reflux disease. *Gut.* 1991;32(2):128–132.

23. Bernstein LM BL. A clinical test for esophagitis. *Gastroenterology.* 1958;34: 760–781.

24. Richter JE, Hewson EG, Sinclair JW, Dalton CB. Acid perfusion test and 24-hour esophageal pH monitoring with symptom index. Comparison of tests for esophageal acid sensitivity. *Dig Dis Sci.* 1991;36(5):565–571.

25. Mehta AJ, De Caestecker JS, Camm AJ, Northfield TC. Sensitization to painful distention and abnormal sensory perception in the esophagus. *Gastroenterology.* 1995;108(2):311–319.

26. Peghini PL, Johnston BT, Leite LP, Castell DO. Mucosal acid exposure sensitizes a subset of normal subjects to intra-oesophageal balloon distension. *Eur J Gastroenterol Hepatol.* 1996;8(10): 979–983.

27. DeVault KR. Acid infusion does not affect intraesophageal balloon distention-induced sensory and pain thresholds. *Am J Gastroenterol.* 1997;92(6):947–949.

28. Sarkar S, Aziz Q, Woolf CJ, Hobson AR, Thompson DG. Contribution of central sensitisation to the development of non-cardiac chest pain. *Lancet.* 2000; 356(9236):1154–1159.

29. Sarkar S, Hobson AR, Hughes A, et al. The prostaglandin E2 receptor-1 (EP-1) mediates acid-induced visceral pain hypersensitivity in humans. *Gastroenterology.* 2003;124(1):18–25.

30. Willert RP, Woolf CJ, Hobson AR, Delaney C, Thompson DG, Aziz Q. The development and maintenance of human visceral pain hypersensitivity is dependent on the

N-methyl-D-aspartate receptor. *Gastroenterology*. 2004;126(3):683-692.

31. Willert R. *Receptor Mechanisms Mediating Human Oesophageal Hypersensitivity* [dissertation]. Manchester: University of Manchester; 2005.

32. Tougas G, Spaziani R, Hollerbach S, et al. Cardiac autonomic function and oesophageal acid sensitivity in patients with non-cardiac chest pain. *Gut*. 2001;49(5): 706-712.

33. Hollerbach S, Bulat R, May A, et al. Abnormal cerebral processing of oesophageal stimuli in patients with noncardiac chest pain (NCCP). *Neurogastroenterol Motil*. 2000;12(6):555-565.

34. Chen CL, Orr WC. Autonomic responses to heartburn induced by esophageal acid infusion. *J Gastroenterol Hepatol*. 2004; 19(8):922-926.

35. Lee YC, Wang HP, Lin LY, Lee BC, Chiu HM, Wu MS, et al. Heart rate variability in patients with different manifestations of gastroesophageal reflux disease. *Auton Neurosci*. 2004;116(1-2):39-45.

36. Drewes AM, Schipper KP, Dimcevski G, et al. Multi-modal induction and assessment of allodynia and hyperalgesia in the human oesophagus. *Eur J Pain*. 2003; 7(6):539-549.

37. Pedersen J, Reddy H, Funch-Jensen P, Arendt-Nielsen L, Gregersen H, Drewes AM. Cold and heat pain assessment of the human oesophagus after experimental sensitisation with acid. *Pain*. 2004; 110(1-2):393-399.

38. Szallasi A, Blumberg PM. Vanilloid (Capsaicin) receptors and mechanisms. *Pharmacol Rev*. 1999;51(2):159-212.

39. Sterner O, Szallasi A. Novel natural vanilloid receptor agonists: new therapeutic targets for drug development. *Trends Pharmacol Sci*. 1999;20(11):459-465.

40. Matthews PJ, Aziz Q, Facer P, Davis JB, Thompson DG, Anand P. Increased capsaicin receptor TRPV1 nerve fibres in the inflamed human oesophagus. *Eur J Gastroenterol Hepatol*. 2004;16(9):897-902.

41. Ciganek L. The EEG response (evoked potential) to light stimulus in man. *Electroenceph Clin Neurophysiol*. 1961;13: 163-172.

42. Desmedt JE. Somatosensory CEP in man. In: Cobb WA, ed. *Handbook of Electroencephalography and Neurophysiology*. Amsterdam: Elsevier;1971:55-82.

43. Giesler CD, Frishkopf LS, Rosenblith WA. Extracranial response to acoustic clicks in man. *Science*. 1958;128:108-121.

44. Hobson AR, Sarkar S, Furlong PL, Thompson DG, Aziz Q. A cortical evoked potential study of afferents mediating human esophageal sensation. *Am J Physiol Gastrointest Liver Physiol*. 2000;279(1): G139-G147.

45. Hollerbach S, Hudoba P, Fitzpatrick D, Hunt R, Upton AR, Tougas G. Cortical evoked responses following esophageal balloon distension and electrical stimulation in healthy volunteers. *Dig Dis Sci*. 1998;43(11):2558-2566.

46. Smout AJ, DeVore MS, Dalton CB, Castell DO. Cerebral potentials evoked by oesophageal distension in patients with non-cardiac chest pain. *Gut*. 1992;33(3): 298-302.

47. Frobert O, Arendt Nielsen L, Bak P, Funch Jensen P, Peder Bagger J. Pain perception and brain evoked potentials in patients with angina despite normal coronary angiograms. *Heart*. 1996;75(5):436-441.

48. Sarkar S, Hobson AR, Furlong PL, Woolf CJ, Thompson DG, Aziz Q. Central neural mechanisms mediating human visceral hypersensitivity. *Am J Physiol Gastrointest Liver Physiol*. 2001;281(5):G1196-G1202.

49. Hobson AR, Aziz Q. Brain imaging and functional gastrointestinal disorders: has it helped our understanding? *Gut*. 2004; 53(8):1198-1206.

50. Hobson AR, Furlong PL, Sarkar S, et al. Neurophysiologic assessment of esophageal sensory processing in noncardiac chest pain. *Gastroenterology*. 2006; 130(1):80-88.

CHAPTER 6

Psychological Disorders and Noncardiac Chest Pain

Guy D. Eslick

Introduction

Historically, the relationship between various psychological disorders and noncardiac chest pain date back to the nineteenth century. Since the early descriptions of "soldiers heart" in the 1860s,[1-4] there have been many descriptions of chest pain syndromes associated with anxiety disorders. In the 1860s the term "soldier's heart" (or irritable heart) was used to describe British soldiers who, during the Crimean War, presented with chest pain or other symptoms of a possible cardiac etiology (Fig 6-1).[5-11] Jacob DaCosta (1871)[3] (Fig 6-2) observed a similar syndrome during the U.S. Civil War and postulated that the "irritable heart" was caused by disordered innervation, very similar to the concept of altered visceral nociception.[12]

Early Work and Associated Disorders

The first large published study assessing psychological disorders and chest pain found that soldiers ($n = 200$) with recurrent chest pain had a high prevalence of acute anxiety (17%), chronic anxiety state (14%), psychopathic personality (18%), depression (12%), and hysteria (11%).[13] Over the last three decades there has been a burgeoning body of literature and evidence supporting a psychological association with noncardiac chest pain. Indeed, numerous psychological conditions have been investigated and associated with noncardiac chest pain; these include panic disorder, generalized anxiety disorder, phobic disorder, major depression, obsessive-compulsive disorder, and somatization.[14-20] In addition,

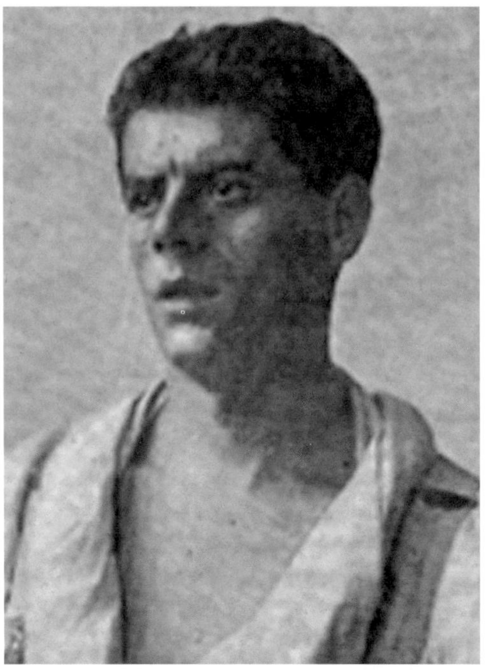

Fig 6–1. A 28-year-old patient with a face typical of "DAH" (disordered action of the heart), one of the many terms used to describe soldier's heart. The picture was taken after 15 minutes of general exercise, and shows dilated nostrils, furrowed forehead, slightly opened mouth, and the general expression of fatigue and anxiety. These features were common to the description of both DAH and soldier's heart, and were given special attention as usual diagnostic features. (From Lewis T. The tolerance of physical exertion as shown by soldier's suffering from so-called "irritable heart." *British Medical Journal* 1918;364).

almost 75% of patients with "near normal" coronary arteries reportedly have some form of psychiatric diagnosis.[21] However, the high levels of apparent psychiatric morbidity may be related to referral bias or alternatively fear of serious disease at the time of the psychiatric assessment.

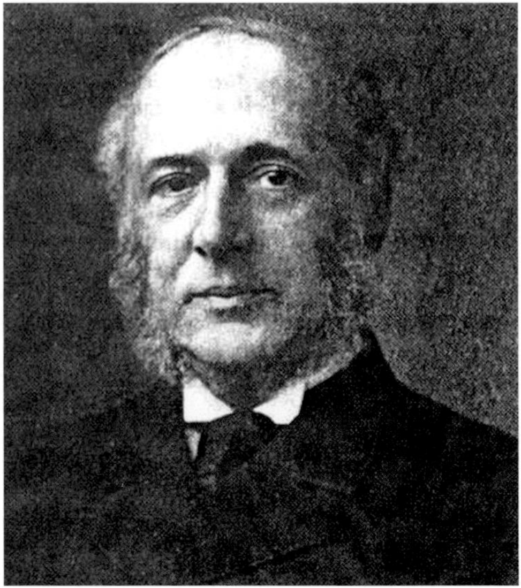

Fig 6–2. Jacob DaCosta. (From Wooley CF. Jacob Mendez DaCosta: Medical teacher, clinician, and clinical investigator. *American Journal of Cardiology.* 1982;50: 1145-1148.)

Current Studies

The majority of studies are hospital-based with only two population-based studies[22,23] providing data linking psychological disorders to noncardiac chest pain. One study assessed the relationships between psychosocial and developmental antecedents of chest pain among a cohort ($n = 3322/5362$) of subjects aged 36 years.[24] The study reported that chest pain (in particular exertional chest pain) was strongly associated (OR: 29.08, 95% CI: 6.65–127.15) with psychiatric disorder; childhood experiences including parental illness were associated with subsequent chest pain.[24] However, there were limitations to this study: first, the strong association was based on a sample of only 32 cases with exertional chest pain (hence a wide confidence interval); second, a family history of heart disease (among some of the participant's fathers) and the inherent potential for recall bias due to the age of the subjects; and last, it was also not possible to screen all subjects for chest pain due to coronary artery disease.

The first community-based study that assessed noncardiac chest pain and psychological disorders was conducted in Australia on a random sample of 1,000 residents in Sydney who were mailed a validated self-report questionnaire.[22] There were three psychological disorders measured which included anxiety, depression, and neuroticism, which were assessed using the validated Hospital Anxiety and Depression Scale (HADS) and the Eysenck Personality Questionnaire (EPQ). The response rate was 73% (n = 672; mean age 46 years; 52% female). Over one third of the population (33%) were classified as having noncardiac chest pain. The prevalence of clinical depression was 7% (95% CI: 4–11%) and anxiety 23% (95% CI: 18–29%) among those with noncardiac chest pain. The authors found that those reporting noncardiac chest pain compared to those with nil pain had significantly higher rates of neuroticism (OR: 1.14, 95% CI: 1.08–1.21), and anxiety (OR: 1.12, 95% CI: 1.08–1.17) but not depression (OR: 1.05, 95% CI: 0.99–1.10). Moreover, the mean scores were higher in those with severe noncardiac chest pain compared to those with mild noncardiac chest pain for neuroticism (OR: 1.16, 95% CI: 1.02–1.31), anxiety (OR: 1.13, 95% CI: 1.03–1.24), and depression (OR: 1.12, 95% CI: 1.01–1.23). The second population-based study was a telephone survey of 2,209 ethnic Hong Kong Chinese households to study the epidemiology of noncardiac chest pain. The telephone interviews were carried out using the Rose Angina Questionnaire, a validated gastroesophageal reflux disease (GERD) questionnaire, and the Hospital Anxiety-Depression Scale. The study reported that those with noncardiac chest pain had significantly higher anxiety (p <0.001) and depression score (p = 0.007), than subjects with no chest pain.

The bulk of the literature in terms of the types of psychological disorders associated with noncardiac chest pain has focused on panic attacks.[14,16,20,25–33] Only a few studies have ascertained the relationship between depression and chest pain,[27,29] which is perplexing as there is considerable overlap between panic disorder and depression.[34] Moreover, there are very few studies that have assessed pathophysiologic aspects linking panic disorder to chest pain symptoms.[35,36]

Some studies have specifically aimed to determine the prevalence of depression and chest pain.[27,29] The first study consisted of 104 atypical or nonanginal chest pain patients attending a cardiology clinic who were assessed based on a structured clinical interview (DSM-III).[27] Almost half (41%) of those without coronary artery disease (n = 43) met the diagnostic criteria for panic disorder, whereas 44% (n = 19) had suffered depression during their lifetime (21% current, 23% past). Furthermore, the study found that females with noncardiac chest pain aged less than 43 years were the most likely group to have panic disorder. The authors felt that the combination of panic disorder and depression among chest pain patients may make successful treatment and resolution of chest pain symptoms more difficult, compared with having a single psychological disorder. The second study evaluated 229 of 334 (69%) acute chest pain patients that presented to a hospital emergency department for assessment of their symptoms.[29] Psychological status was determined by an interview questionnaire (consisting of the Panic Disorder Self-Rating Scale (PDSRS), Beck Anxiety Inventory (BDI), and the Zung Self-Rating Anxiety Scale (SAS) within 48 hours of admission. The prevalence of panic disorder and depression was 17.5% and 23.1%, respectively, but controls were not evaluated.

The prevalence of panic disorder in the population is approximately 1 to 2%.[37] Most studies of panic disorder patients have focused on patients presenting for psychiatric or psychological treatments. More recently, the focus of this research has turned to medical populations, in particular, individuals presenting with chest pain to the Emergency Department, because more than two-thirds suffer from anxiety/panic disorder with no sign of organic disease.[38] Furthermore, one study has reported that panic disorder is a rarely recognized condition among patients presenting with chest pain (8%, $n = 4/51$) to family physicians.[26] The criteria for panic attack (DSM-IV) are shown below.

Criteria for Panic Attack (DSM-IV)

A discrete period of intense fear or discomfort, in which four (or more) of the following symptoms developed abruptly and reached a peak within 10 minutes.

- Palpitations, pounding heart, or accelerated heart rate
- Sweating
- Trembling or shaking
- Sensations of shortness of breath or smothering
- Feeling of choking
- Chest pain or discomfort
- Nausea or abdominal distress
- Feeling dizzy, unsteady, light-headed, or faint
- Derealization (feeling of unreality) or depersonalization (being detached from oneself)
- Fear of losing control or going crazy
- Fear of dying
- Paresthesias (numbness or tingling sensations)
- Chills or hot flushes

Chest pain is a common symptom in people having panic attacks.[16,39] Moreover, several well-designed studies that have investigated the impact of panic disorder among those with noncardiac chest pain have reported the prevalence of panic disorder is between 15% to 70%.[16,20,39-42] The majority of these studies report that, in terms of predictors of panic disorder, noncardiac chest pain tends to be more common in younger women (<30 years of age) with chest pain and no family history of heart disease.[42] It should be remembered that although not all patients can be profiled in this way the presence of these predictors in patients with acute chest pain should certainly increase the index of suspicion for panic disorder as a cause of chest pain.

There are conflicting reports regarding the association between esophageal abnormalities and psychiatric disease. In patients with chest pain, psychiatric disorders can overlap with esophageal disease. One study found that in a group of patients with motor abnormalities of the esophagus, over 80% also had a psychiatric disorder.[43] In contrast, another study reported less than one-third of patients with normal esophageal motility were found to have a psychiatric abnormality.[44]

Potential Mechanisms

In the situation where there is overlap between the psychological state of the patient and physical disease, it is uncertain which is the primary event.[19] It may be that the psychiatric disorder is the primary pathology and that the visceral abnormality is brought on and exacerbated by the underlying psychological state of the patient. Lower thresholds for pain following balloon distension of the esophagus[45] and altered central nervous system responses to visceral stimuli occur in patients with noncardiac chest pain.[46] Possibly because tricyclic antidepressants

have local as well as central analgesic actions,[47] this class of drugs have had encouraging results in patients with noncardiac chest pain.[48]

It has been postulated that the high prevalence of psychiatric morbidity in patients with chest pain and normal coronary arteries indicates that the pain is multifactorial in origin (Fig 6–3).[50] There have been several psychosocial factors associated with noncardiac chest pain. Treatment of the psychological comorbidity aspect of the disease may be as important as treatment of any underlying structural disorder. Coulshed and Eslick[51] suggested the importance of providing a diagnostic "label" for patients with noncardiac chest pain to reduce underlying patient anxiety. In addition, comprehensive testing for esophageal disorders with or without psychiatric abnormalities is clearly a major undertaking, and an alternative remains empiric

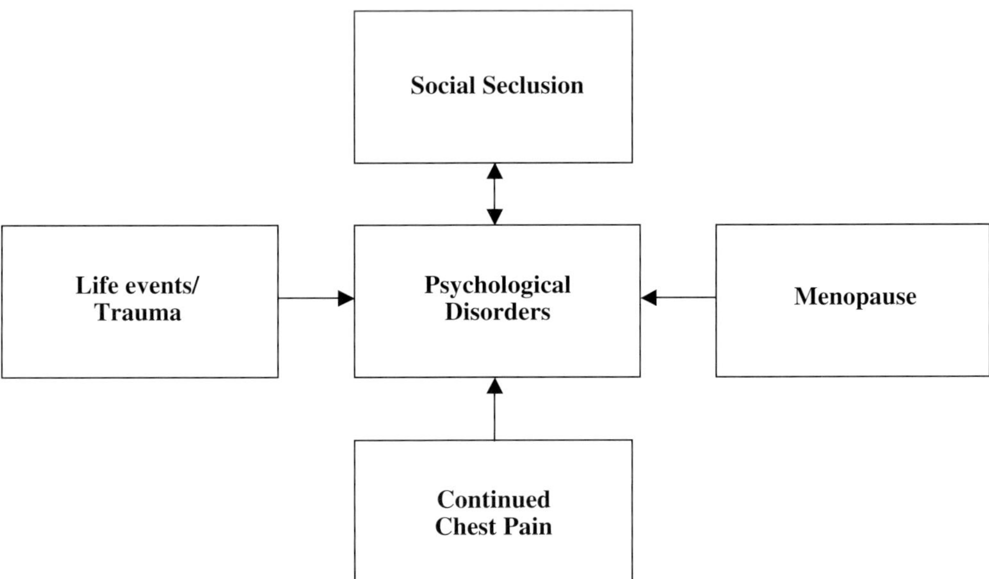

Fig 6–3. Interplay between factors related to psychological disorders and noncardiac chest pain (adapted from Asbury & Collins[49]).

treatment with other drug groups (eg, calcium channel blockers or tricyclics); this may be a more practical and less costly approach.[52] However, in a recent review article the authors recommended a new treatment tactic in terms of psychological treatments for those with noncardiac chest pain in the Emergency Department or outpatient setting.[53] The suggested proposal involves using the biopsychosocial model which incorporates most often cognitive behavioral therapy (CBT), with the main aim of decreasing the frequency, severity, and distress of physical symptoms (ie, chest pain).

Children and Adolescents

Lipsitz et al[54] conducted a study of 27 young people aged 8 to 17 years with noncardiac chest pain after assessment by a pediatric cardiologist. The study found that almost two-thirds (59%) were classified as having a psychological disorder according to the DSM-IV. Furthermore, over half (56%) of the individuals had an anxiety disorder, with 60% of these diagnosed with panic disorder. Only one individual had a depressive disorder. The authors concluded that anxiety was a common psychological disorder linked with noncardiac chest pain among children and adolescents.

Summary

It should be noted that many of the studies in the early literature are lacking in terms of methodologic rigor.[13] Indeed, many of these studies had no control groups and also no standardized instruments or measures were used in assessing the psychological disorders in question, rather, subjective observations were the basis of a psychiatric diagnosis in these studies.[13] Over the last decade, there has been a large increase in the number of psychometric scales developed for use in medical research.[55] Furthermore, the ability to compare normal controls to patients with chest pain of noncardiac origin in terms of their psychological differences in a standardized and validated manner represents an immense improvement in our ability to investigate the psychological substrates of noncardiac chest pain. This improvement can be most strongly associated with the development of standardized psychiatric diagnostic criteria in the form of the *Diagnostic and Statistical Manual of the American Psychiatric Association* (DSM-IV). This has provided a more robust classification of the psychiatric disorders that have been associated with noncardiac chest pain such as panic disorder, generalized anxiety disorders, obsessive-compulsive disorders, depression, and somatoform disorders. Further research is needed is this area, with emphasis on development of simple screening tools within emergency departments and new therapeutic treatments for those with recalcitrant noncardiac chest pain.

References

1. MacLean WC. Diseases of the heart in the British Army: the cause and the remedy. *Brit Med J.* 1867;i:161–164.
2. Myers ABR. *On the Etiology and Prevalence of Diseases of the Heart among Soldiers.* London: J Churchill; 1870.

3. DaCosta JM. On irritable heart. *Am J Med Sci*. 1871;61:17-52.
4. Beard G. Neurasthenia, or nervous exhaustion. *Boston Med Surg J*. 1869;III: 217-221.
5. Jarcho S. Functional heart disease in the Civil War (DaCosta 1871). *Am J Cardiol*. 1959;4:809-817.
6. Howell JD. "Soldier's heart": The redefinition of heart disease and speciality formation in early twentieth-century Great Britain. *Med History*. 1985;5:34-52.
7. Wood P. Da Costa's syndrome (or effort syndrome): the mechanism of the somatic manifestations. *Brit Med J*. 1941a;May 31: 805-811.
8. Wood P. Aetiology of DaCosta's syndrome. *Brit Med J*. 1941b;June7:845-851.
9. Wooley CF. From irritable heart to mitral valve prolapse: British army medical reports, 1860 to 1870. *Am J Cardiol*. 1985; 55:1107-1109.
10. Wooley CF. From irritable heart to mitral valve prolapse: World War I—the U.S. experience and the origin of neurocirculatory asthenia. *Am J Cardiol*. 1987;59: 1183-1186.
11. Wooley CF. Jacob Mendez DaCosta: Medical teacher, clinician, and clinical investigator. *Am J Cardiol*. 1982;50:1145-1148.
12. Cannon RO 3rd. The gastroenterologist and microvascular angina. *Gastroenterology*. 1990;98:1103-1105.
13. Jones M, Lewis A. Effort syndrome. *Lancet*. 1941;June 28;813-818.
14. Potokar JP, Nutt DJ. Chest pain: panic attack or heart attack? *Int J Clin Pract*. 2000;54:110-114.
15. Okpa K, Morley S, Hobson AR, et al. Psychological responses to episodic chest pain. *Eur J Pain*. 2003;7:521-529.
16. Huffman JC, Pollack MH. Predicting panic disorder among patients with chest pain: an analysis of the literature. *Psychosomatics*. 2003;44:222-236.
17. Alexander PJ, Prabhu SGS, Krishnamoorthy ES, Halkatti PC. Mental disorders in patients with noncardiac chest pain. *Acta Psychiatrica Scandinavica*. 1994; 89:291-293.
18. Carter CS, Maddock RJ. Chest pain in generalized anxiety disorder. *Int J Psychiat Med*. 1992;22:291-298.
19. Clouse RE, Carney RM. The psychological profile of noncardiac chest pain patients. *Eur J Gastroenterol Hepatol*. 1995;7:1160-1165.
20. Dammen T, Ekeberg O, Arnesen H, Friis S. Personality profiles in patients referred for chest pain. Investigation with emphasis on panic disorder patients. *Psychosomatics*. 2000;41:269-276.
21. Bass C, Wade C, Hand D, Jackson G. Patients with angina with normal and near normal coronary arteries: clinical and psychosocial state 12 months after angiography. *Brit Med J*. 1983;287: 1505-1508.
22. Eslick GD, Jones MP, Talley NJ. Non-cardiac chest pain: prevalence, risk factors, impact and consulting—a population-based study. *Aliment Pharmacol Ther*. 2003;17:1115-1124.
23. Wong WM, Lam KF, Cheng C, et al. Population based study of noncardiac chest pain in southern Chinese: prevalence, psychosocial factors and health care utilization. *World J Gastroenterol*. 2004; 10(5):702-712.
24. Hotopf M, Mayou R, Wadsworth M, Wessely S. Psychosocial and developmental antecedents of chest pain in young adults. *Psychosomatic Med*. 1999;61:861-867.
25. Dammen T, Ekeberg O, Arnesen H, Friis S. The detection of panic disorder in chest pain patients. *Gen Hosp Psychiat*. 1999; 21:323-332.
26. Katerndahl DA, Trammell C. Prevalence and recognition of panic states in STARNET patients presenting with chest pain. *J Family Pract*. 1997;45:54-63.
27. Beitman BD, Basha I, Flaker G, DeRosear L, Mukerji V, Trombka L, Katow W. Atypical or nonanginal chest pain. Panic disorder or coronary artery disease? *Arch Intern Med*. 1987;147:1548-1552.

28. Carter C, Maddock R, Amsterdam E, McCormick S, Waters C, Billett J. Panic disorder and chest pain in the coronary care unit. *Psychosomatics.* 1992;33: 302-309.

29. Yingling KW, Wulsin LR, Arnold LM, Rouan GW. Estimated prevalence of panic disorder and depression among consecutive patients seen in an emergency department with acute chest pain. *J Gen Intern Med.* 1993;8: 231-235.

30. Beitman BD, Mukerji V, Lamberti JW, et al. Panic disorder in patients with chest pain and angiographically normal coronary arteries. *Am J Med.* 1989;63:1399-1403.

31. Beitman BD. Panic disorder in patients with angiographically normal coronary arteries. *Am J Med.* 1992;92(suppl 5A): 33S-40S.

32. Jeejeebhoy FM, Dorian P, Newman DM. Panic disorder and the heart: a cardiology perspective. *J Psychosomatic Res.* 2000;48:393-403.

33. Mansour VM, Wilkinson DJC, Jennings GL, Schwarz RG, Thompson JM, Esler MD. Panic disorder: coronary spasm as a basis for cardiac risk? *Med J Aust.* 1998;168: 390-392.

34. Breier A, Charney DS, Heniger GB. Major depression in patients with agoraphobia and panic disorder. *Arch Gen Psychiat.* 1984;41:1129-1135.

35. Lynch P, Bakal DA, Whitelaw W, Fung T. Chest muscle activity and panic anxiety: a preliminary investigation. *Psychosomatic Med.* 1991;53:80-89.

36. Stollman NH, Bierman PS, Ribiero Al, Rogers AI. CO_2 provocation of panic: symptomatic and manometric evaluation in patients with noncardiac chest pain. *Am J Gastroenterol.* 1997;92:839-842.

37. Weissman MM, Merikangas KR. The epidemiology of anxiety and panic disorders: an update. *J Clin Psychiat.* 1986; 47(suppl):11-17.

38. Demiryoguran NS, Karcioglu O, Topacoglu H, et al. Anxiety disorder in patients with non-specific chest pain in the emergency setting. *Emerg Med J.* 2006;23:99-102.

39. Fleet RP, Dupuis G, Marchand A, Burelle D, Arsnault A, Beitman BD. Panic disorder in emergency department chest pain patients: prevalence, comorbidity, suicidal ideation, and physician recognition. *Am J Med.* 1996;101:371-380.

40. Ho KY, Kang JY, Yeo B, Ng WL. Noncardiac, non-oesophageal chest pain—the relevance of psychological factors. *Gut.* 1998;43:105-110.

41. Maddock RJ, Carter CS, Tavano-Hall L, Amsterdam EA. Hypocapnia associated with cardiac stress scintigraphy in chest pain patients with panic disorder. *Psychosomatic Med.* 1998;60:52-55.

42. Fleet RP, Beitman BD. Unexplained chest pain: when is it panic disorder? *Clin Cardiol.* 1997;20:187-194.

43. Clouse RE, Lustman PJ. Psychiatric illness and contraction abnormalities of the esophagus. *N Engl J Med.* 1983;309: 1337-1342.

44. Kahrilas PJ. Nutcracker esophagus: Editorial: an idea whose time has gone? *Am J Gastroenterol.* 1993;88:167-169.

45. Rao SS, Gregersen H, Hayek B, et al. Noncardiac chest pain: the hypersensitive, hyperreactive, and poorly compliant esophagus. *Ann Intern Med.* 1996;124: 950-958.

46. Frobert O, Funch-Jensen P, Bagger JP. Diagnostic value of esophageal studies in patients with angina-like chest pain and normal coronary angiograms. *Ann Intern Med.* 1996;124:959-969.

47. Cannon RO 3rd, Quyyumi AA, Mincemoyer R, et al. Imipramine in patients with chest pain despite normal coronary angiograms. *N Engl J Med.* 1994;20: 1411-1417.

48. Clouse RE. Antidepressants for functional gastrointestinal syndromes. *Dig Dis Sci.* 1994;39:2352-2363.

49. Asbury, EA, Collins P. Psychosocial factors associated with noncardiac chest pain and cardiac syndrome X. *Herz.* 2005;30 (1):55-60.

50. Potts SG, Bass CM. Psychosocial outcome and use of medical resources in patients with chest pain and normal or near-normal coronary arteries: a long-term follow-up study. *Quart J Med.* 1993;86: 583–593.

51. Coulshed DS, Eslick GD, Talley NJ. Noncardiac chest pain: patients need diagnoses. *Brit Med J.* 2002;324:915.

52. Langdon DE. Empiric therapy for noncardiac chest pain. *Arch Intern Med.* 2000; 160:3331.

53. Esler JL, Bock BC. Psychological treatments for noncardiac chest pain: Recommendations for a new approach. *J Psychosomatic Res.* 2004;56:263–269.

54. Lipsitz JD, Masia C, Apfel H, et al. Noncardiac chest pain and psychopathology in children and adolescents. *J Psychosomatic Res.* 2005;59:185–188.

55. Endenborough R. *Using Psychometrics: A Practical Guide to Testing and Assessment.* 2nd ed. London: Kogan Page; 1999.

CHAPTER 7

Diagnosis of Noncardiac Chest Pain

Elisa M. Faybush
Ronnie Fass

Introduction

The burden of making the diagnosis of noncardiac chest pain (NCCP) is currently placed on the cardiologist as symptoms of NCCP are indistinguishable from those of cardiac angina.[1] Once cardiac cause for chest pain has been excluded, patients are often referred to a gastroenterologist in the hope of uncovering an esophageal abnormality, as the esophagus is the most common source of symptoms in patients with NCCP. It has been estimated that 23 to 80% of subjects with NCCP have some type of esophageal abnormality, which includes GERD and a variety of esophageal motor disorders.[2]

By far, GERD is the most common cause of NCCP, accounting for up to 60% of patients.[3] Among patients with non-GERD related NCCP, up to 30% have an esophageal motor disorder.[4-6] However, 70% of those with non-GERD related NCCP have normal esophageal motility but may demonstrate alteration in esophageal pain perception (visceral hyperalgesia).

Thus, the main esophageal underlying mechanisms for NCCP include GERD, esophageal motility abnormalities and visceral hypersensitivity. This chapter focuses on the currently available diagnostic tests that are used to evaluate for the presence of the underlying mechanisms of NCCP (Table 7-1).

GERD-Related NCCP

There is no gold standard for diagnosing GERD-related NCCP. The currently available diagnostic tests to detect GERD in patients with NCCP include barium swallow, upper endoscopy, the acid perfusion test, ambulatory 24-hour esophageal pH monitoring, and the PPI test.

Table 7–1. Diagnostic Tests for Noncardiac Chest Pain

Gastroesophageal reflux
- Acid perfusion test (Bernstein test)
- Ambulatory 24-hour esophageal pH monitoring
- Barium swallow
- Proton-pump inhibitor (PPI) test
- Upper endoscopy

Esophageal dysmotility
- Bethanechol test
- Esophageal manometry
- Edrophonium (Tensilon) test
- Ergonovine test
- High-frequency intraluminal ultrasonography
- Impedance planimetry
- Pentagastrin test

Visceral hypersensitivity
- Balloon distension test
- Electrical stimulation
- Impedance planimetry
- Brain imaging

Barium Esophagram

Barium esophagram has very little use in the diagnosis of GERD. Barium esophagram has a low sensitivity (20%) for diagnosing GERD in general due to lack of anatomic and mucosal abnormalities in most GERD patients.[7] Furthermore, the significance of barium reflux during the procedure as a diagnostic for GERD is questionable. Johnston et al found that the proportion of patients with an abnormal 24-hour esophageal pH study was similar to the proportion of patients with a normal 24-hour esophageal pH study, who had spontaneous barium reflux during the test.[7] Additionally, spontaneous barium reflux has been demonstrated in up to 20% of healthy subjects.[8]

The role of barium esophagram is even less clear in patients with GERD-related NCCP, primarily due to the rare presence of esophageal mucosal abnormalities. However, one may consider performing a barium esophagram as the initial diagnostic test in patients who report dysphagia in addition to chest pain.

Upper Endoscopy

Once a patient is referred to a gastroenterologist for evaluation of NCCP, if any alarm symptoms (decreased appetite, weight loss, dysphagia, odynophagia, hematemesis, and anemia) are present, an upper endoscopy is warranted to rule out mucosal abnormalities such as benign or malignant tumors, esophageal ulceration, or peptic stricture.

Upper endoscopy is the best test for identifying esophageal mucosal involvement in GERD (erosive esophagitis, stricture, ulcers, and Barrett's esophagus). However, it is not a useful test in the initial evaluation of NCCP because only a small minority of patients (10–25%) will have endoscopic evidence of esophageal mucosal injury.[9]

The diagnostic yield of upper endoscopy, esophageal manometry, and Bernstein testing was assessed in 100 consecutive patients being evaluated for NCCP. Upper endoscopy revealed grade II to IV esophagitis in only 24 patients (24%).[10] Frobert et al[11] investigated the clinical value of upper endoscopy in NCCP and found that only 15 (31%) of the patients had esophageal mucosal injury, with all but one having grade I erosive esophagitis.

Interestingly, despite lack of evidence to support the usage of upper endoscopy as the initial test in the evaluation of NCCP, it is the most commonly used diagnostic modality in clinical practice.[12]

Acid Perfusion Test

In 1958, Bernstein and Baker described the acid perfusion test as a reliable method for the reproduction of esophageal pain (Fig 7-1).[13] The acid perfusion test was originally performed in a fasting patient sitting upright in a chair. A nasogastric tube was placed 30 to 35 cm from the nares so that the acid solution would have been delivered to the midesophagus. The tube was connected to an intravenous bottle. Normal saline was initially administered as a control for 10 to 15 minutes at a rate of 7 to 7.5 mL/minute. This was followed by an infusion of 0.1N HCl at a similar rate for 30 minutes or until chest pain was induced. The test was considered "positive related" if HCl perfusion reproduced patients typical chest pain. When acid induced only a retrosternal burning or other sensations, the test was called "positive unrelated" and was not accepted as proof that acid is the underlying cause of patients chest pain.[14] Over the years, however, many modifications have been made to the acid perfusion test including performing the procedure in the supine position and alteration in the rate and duration of the acid perfusion.

The exact etiology of symptoms during the acid perfusion test remains controversial. Some authorities suggested that

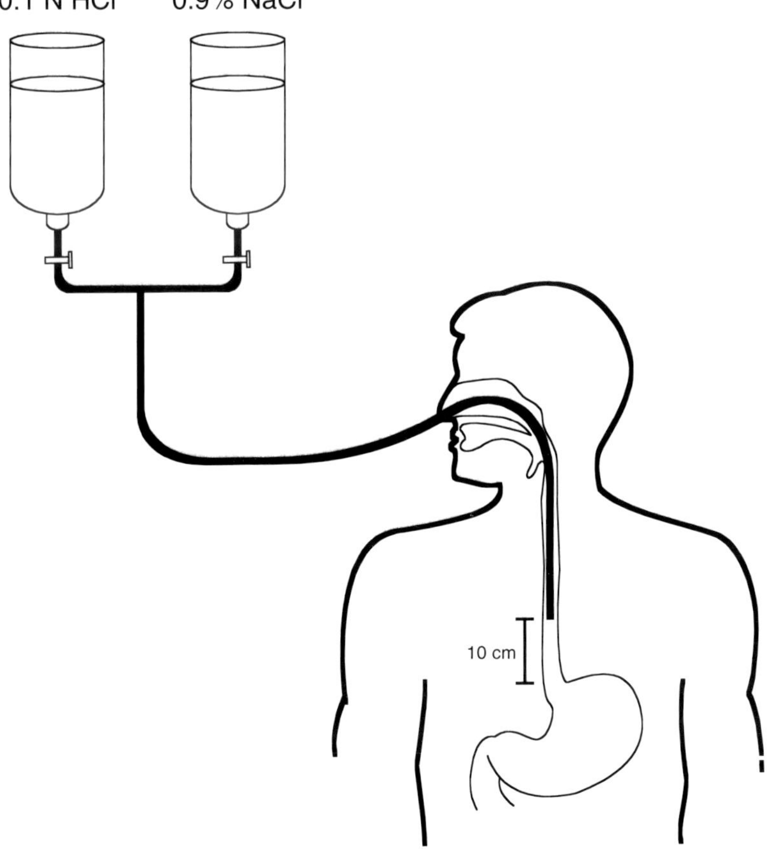

Fig 7–1. The acid perfusion test.

symptoms were attributed to acid-induced esophageal spasm, contact of acid with morphologically damaged esophageal mucosa, increased chemoreceptor sensitivity to acid, or sustained longitudinal muscle contractions.[15,16] Many attempts have been made to change the test from a qualitative to a quantitative tool. Fass et al evaluated chemoreceptor sensitivity to intraluminal acid in patients with mild-to-moderate gastroesophageal reflux disease.[17] A manometry catheter was placed 10 cm above the upper border of the lower esophageal sphincter (LES). Saline was infused initially for 2 minutes and then, without patient's awareness, 1N HCl was infused for 10 minutes at a rate of 10 mL per minute using a dual chamber Harvard apparatus (Fig 7–2). Patients were instructed to report whenever their typical symptoms were reproduced. Esophageal chemosensitivity to acid was assessed by both the duration until typical symptoms were reproduced (expressed in seconds), and the total sensory intensity rating reported by the subject at the end of the acid perfusion, by using a verbal descriptor scale (Fig 7–3). The scale consisted of a 20-cm vertical bar flanked by descriptors of increasing intensity (no sensation, fair, very weak, weak, very mild, moderate, barely strong, slightly intense, strong, intense, very intense, and extremely intense). Placement of words along the side of the scale was determined from their relative log intensity rating in a normative study.[18] An acid perfusion test sensitivity (APSS) score was then calculated from the duration of symptom perception and intensity grading at the conclusion of the test.

The original acid perfusion test is highly specific for GERD-related NCCP, but the sensitivity is relatively low, ranging from 6 to 60%. In a study by Katz et al, only 61 of 910 patients (6.7%) with NCCP had their chest pain reproduced during the acid perfusion test.[6] However, the Bernstein test is relatively inexpensive and easy to perform but presently is rarely used in clinical practice because of its limited diagnostic value in NCCP and the emergence of the proton pump inhibitor test (PPI test).

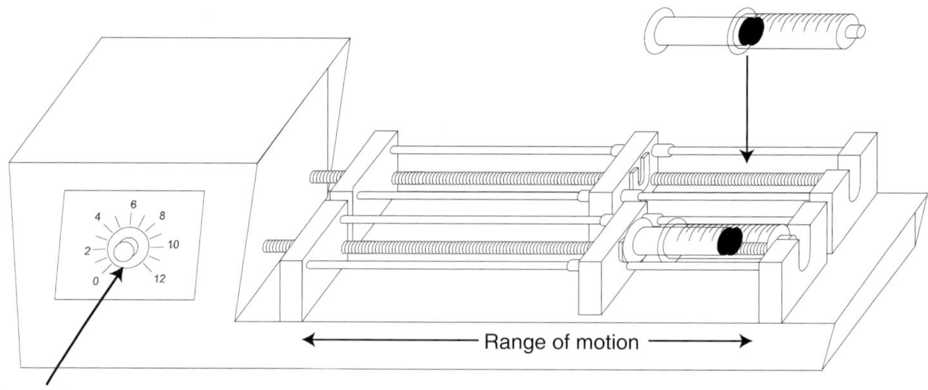

Fig 7–2. A dual chamber infusion pump (Harvard apparatus) used for the acid perfusion test.

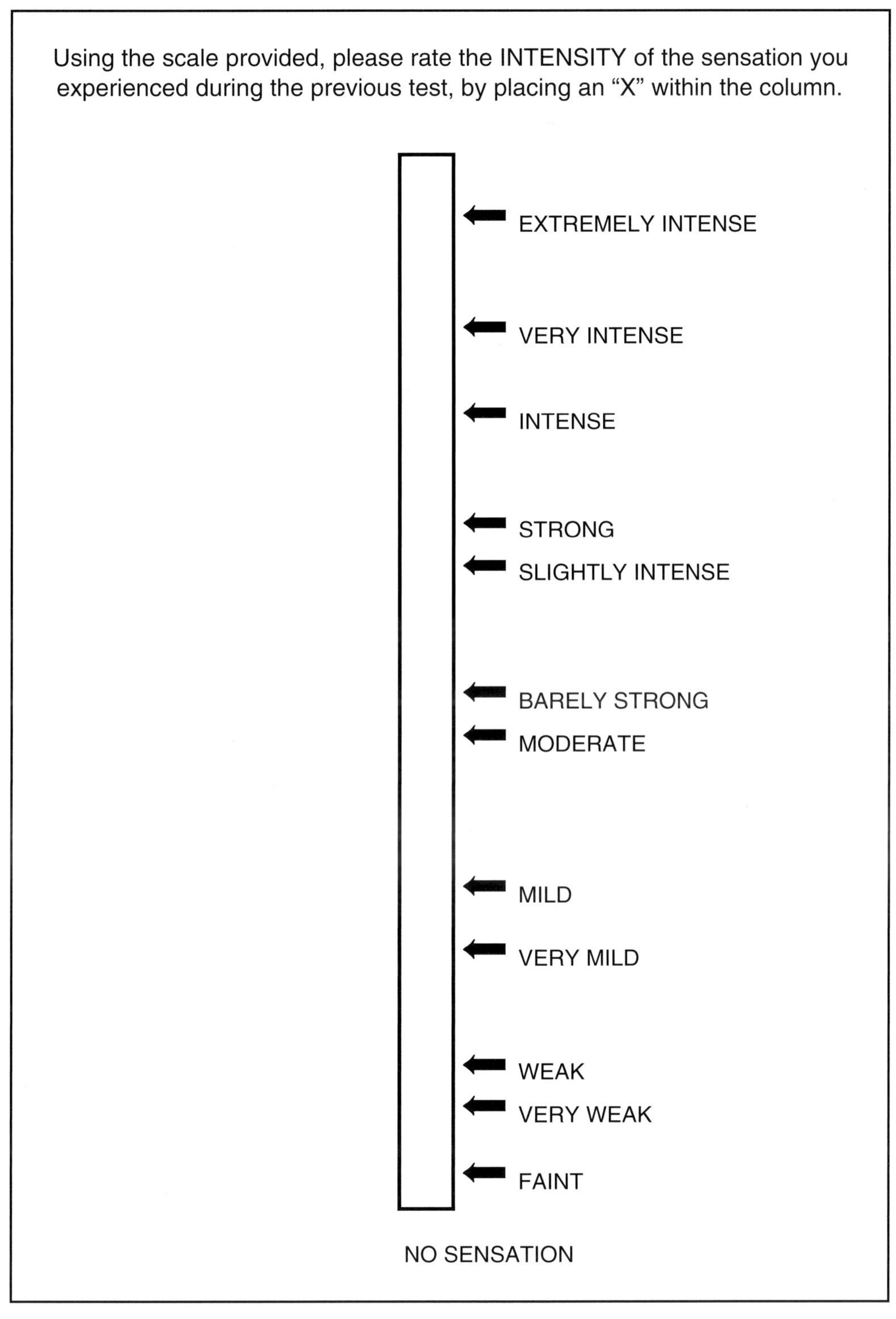

Fig 7–3. A verbal descriptor scale used to assess symptom intensity in patients undergoing the acid perfusion test.[18]

Ambulatory 24-hour Esophageal pH Monitoring

Ambulatory 24-hour esophageal pH monitoring with symptom correlation is still commonly used to evaluate patients with NCCP.[19] Approximately 50 to 60% of NCCP patients have abnormal esophageal acid exposure or a positive symptom index alone. However, the presence of abnormal distal esophageal acid exposure during pH testing does not necessarily mean that the patient's chest pain is GERD related. Hewson et al[19] examined 100 consecutive patients with NCCP and detected abnormal acid exposure in 48% of patients. Of the 83 patients who had spontaneous chest pain during the study, 37 (46%) had abnormal reflux parameters, and 50 (60%) had a normal study but a positive symptom index (calculated as the percentage of symptoms that are associated with acid reflux events). The authors concluded that 24-hour esophageal pH testing with symptom index (SI) is the single best test for evaluating patients with NCCP (Fig 7-4). In contrast, Dekel et al[20] demonstrated that a positive SI is a relatively uncommon phenomenon in NCCP patients because most of the patients do not experience chest pain during the pH study.

The pH test is invasive, inconvenient to patients, costly, and not readily available for many physicians. Additionally, the yield of the test in NCCP has not been rigorously assessed. This is compounded by the rarity of chest pain symptoms during the test in many patients, making it difficult to determine the relationship between patients' symptoms and acid reflux events.[21]

The Wireless pH System

The wireless (Bravo pH system, Medtronic, Shoreview, Minn) pH-monitoring system is a new USFDA class II approved "catheterless" pH monitoring system (Fig 7-5). It involves the attachment of a radiotelemetry pH capsule to the wall of the esophagus (peroral or transnasal). It simultaneously measures pH and transmits data to a pager-sized receiver clipped onto the patient's belt thereby circumventing the need for a nasally placed pH catheter, which is uncomfortable for many patients.[22] Unlike the traditional pH catheter system, the wireless pH system can collect data for up to 48 hours. The system was found to be well tolerated and reliable, and it provided reproducible results.[23] It is a viable alternative for patients unwilling or unable to undergo a conventional ambulatory pH study.

The wireless pH system may prove to be helpful in further clarifying the role of GERD in NCCP and in better determining the relationship between symptoms and acid reflux events in these patients. A recent study by Prakash et al[24] demonstrated that by extending the pH recording period to 48 hours with the wireless pH system in patients with NCCP there was an increase in the number of chest pains reported, resulting in better assessment of the relationship between symptoms and acid reflux events.

The PPI Test

The ideal therapeutic modality for NCCP would combine its evaluation and treatment in a single step. Consequently, the PPI test has become an attractive,

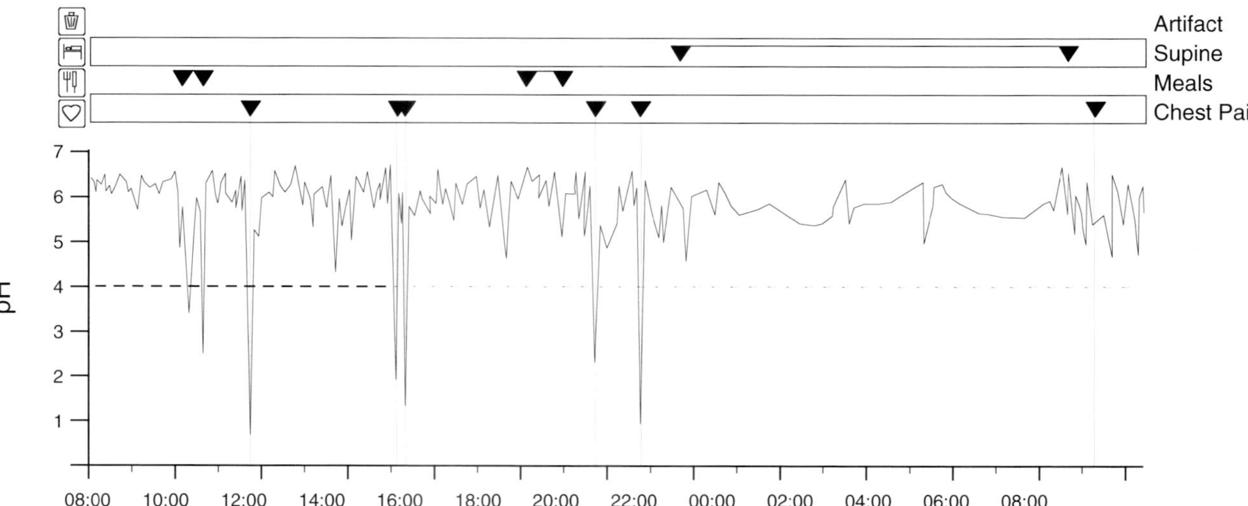

Fig 7–4. A 24-hour pH strip of a patient with NCCP. Of the 6 reported episodes of chest pain during the test, 5 correlated with acid reflux events (SI = 83%).

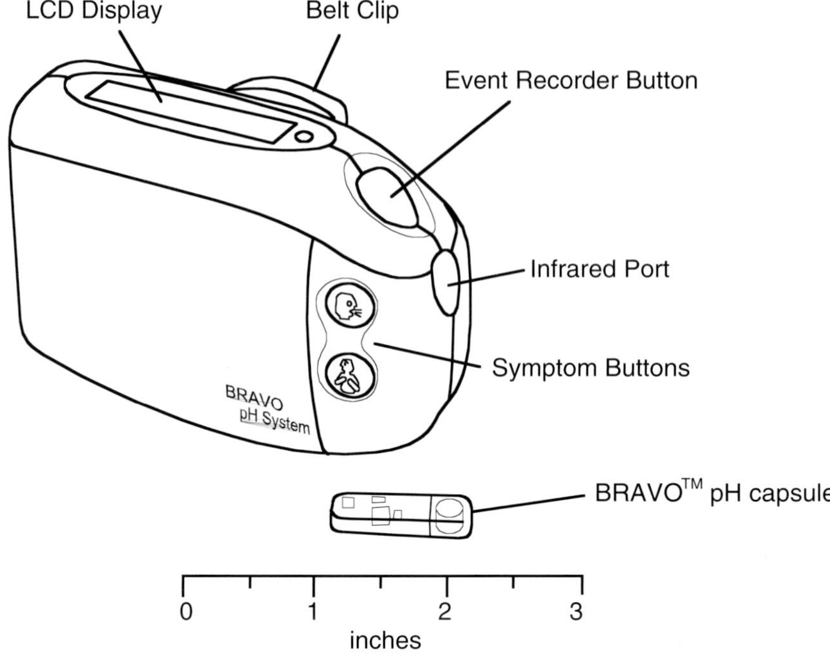

Fig 7–5. A schematic presentation of the wireless pH capsule and the data recorder device.

alternative diagnostic tool for GERD-related NCCP. The test is simple, noninvasive, and at the disposal of primary care physicians and specialists alike. The PPI test uses a short course of high-dose PPI to diagnosis GERD in patients with NCCP. The main objective of the PPI test is to achieve a significant improvement of symptoms in as many patients with GERD-related NCCP as possible within a short period of time.[25] PPIs were selected for the test because of their specific, profound, and consistent inhibitory effect on acid secretion and the marked symptom improvement that they provide to GERD patients.

There have been a number of studies that assessed the diagnostic accuracy of the PPI test in NCCP patients (Table 7–2).[12,26-31] Fass et al used the omeprazole test (40 mg AM and 20 mg PM over a period of 7 days) and found a sensitivity of 78.3% as well as a specificity of 85.7% for diagnosing GERD-related NCCP.[12] The positive predictive value of the omeprazole test was 90%, and the negative predictive value was 70.6%. Other studies have since shown that rabeprazole and lansoprazole are also useful in diagnosing GERD-related NCCP.[29,30]

The use of the PPI test is highly dependent on the frequency of chest pain symptoms. If symptoms occur less than once a week, then the test may be extended to 2 weeks or longer. Studies have demonstrated that the PPI test as the first diagnostic tool in patients with NCCP is a cost-effective strategy. Economic analyses demonstrated that the PPI test saves $573 per average NCCP patient. It also resulted in an 81% reduction in the number of performed endoscopies and a 79% reduction in the usage of 24-hour esophageal pH monitoring.[12]

Table 7–2. Proton-Pump Inhibitor Therapeutic Trials in NCCP

First Author	Reference	Dosing Schedule	No. of Patients	Symptom Improve-ment (%)	Sensitivity (%)	Specificity (%)
Young	(26)	Omeprazole 80 mg/day × 1 day	30	75	90	80
Squillace	(27)	Omeprazole 80 mg/day × 1 day	17	50	69	75
Xia	(30)	Lansoprazole 30 mg/day for 4 weeks	68	50	92	67
Pandak	(31)	Omeprazole 40 mg twice daily × 2 weeks	37	50	90	67
Fass	(12)	Omeprazole (40 mg in the morning and 20 mg in the evening) for 7 days	37	50	78	86
Fass	(28)	Lansoprazole (60 mg in the morning and 30 mg in the evening) for 7 days	40	50	78	82
Fass	(29)	Rabeprazole (20 mg in the morning and 20 mg in the evening) for 7 days	20	50	83	75

Ofman et al[32] performed a decision analysis to evaluate the clinical and economic outcomes of different diagnostic strategies for NCCP comparing an initial trial of the omeprazole test followed by traditional diagnostic strategies (pH testing, endoscopy, and esophageal manometry) versus only traditional diagnostic strategies ordered first in different sequences. Strategies that initially used the PPI test resulted in 84% of the patients being asymptomatic at 1 year compared with 74% for the strategies that began with traditional diagnostic testing. The usage of the PPI test followed by pH testing, endoscopy, and esophageal manometry led to an 11% improvement in diagnostic accuracy and 43% reduction in the use of invasive diagnostic tests.[32]

Multichannel Intraluminal Impedance

Recent introduction of improved impedance probes with integrated pH sensors allowed further assessment of refluxate composition and its relationship to symptoms.[33] Because the electrical conductivity of the esophageal muscular wall, air, and any given bolus is different, the presence of different substances in the esophageal lumen provides a different impedance pattern.[33] With a highly conductive bolus (eg, saliva), the impedance decreases; with poorly conductive material (eg, air), the impedance increases.

The combination of an impedance catheter and a pH probe provides a unique opportunity to study physiologic and pathologic events within the esophagus and their relationship to symptoms. In addition, the recording assembly can disclose the characteristics of the gastric refluxate (acid, nonacid, gas, and mixed gas and liquid). The value of such technique has been demonstrated by recent studies in patients who failed PPIs twice daily, showing that nonacidic reflux is not uncommon in PPI-failure patients and may lead to classic heartburn symptoms as well.[33]

It is apparent that the esophageal impedance technique needs to be standardized and that further studies are required to determine its proper clinical utility specifically in GERD-related NCCP. However, future use of this unique technique may further expand our understanding of symptom generation in these patients and may better direct therapy.

Esophageal Dysmotility

In approximately a third of the patients with non-GERD-related NCCP, various esophageal motility abnormalities have been described.[5,6,34] Thus, in NCCP, esophageal manometry is commonly performed if GERD has been excluded as the underlying cause.[35] The role of esophageal manometry in NCCP has evolved over the last few years, primarily due to lack of effective treatment for the various esophageal motility abnormalities. This was compounded by clinical evidence that patients with non-GERD-related NCCP reported symptom improvement on pain modulators regardless if esophageal dysmotility was present or absent (except for achalasia).[36] Consequently, the role of esophageal manometry in non-GERD-related NCCP appears to be limited to identifying the small number of patients with achalasia.[37]

Esophageal Manometry

Esophageal manometry is the best tool to detect motility disorders of the esophagus. Evaluation of the amplitude of the esophageal contraction wave, its configuration, and propagation as well as the function of the upper and lower esophageal sphincters may be provided.[38]

The relationship between motility abnormalities diagnosed in NCCP patients and chest pain remains controversial. In a large retrospective study of patients with NCCP, only 28% were found to have esophageal dysmotility during esophageal manometry.[6] Nutcracker esophagus was the most common motility disorder (48%) followed by nonspecific esophageal motility disorder (36%), diffuse esophageal spasm (10%), hypertensive LES (4%), and achalasia (2%) (Fig 7–6).

In NCCP patients with esophageal dysmotility, some have stipulated that esophageal spasm, for example, may be the cause of chest pain either by distending the proximal segment of the esophagus (leading to activation of mechanoreceptors) or by producing myoischemia (activation of chemoreceptors).[4] However, in patients with NCCP, documented esophageal manometry abnormalities are rarely associated with symptoms. Therefore, some have suggested that perhaps these abnormalities are not the direct cause of patients' chest pain but rather a marker of an underlying motor disorder.[39] Consequently, documenting the presence of an esophageal motility disorder during esophageal manometry (except achalasia) does not conclusively prove that it is the underlying cause of patients' chest pain. This should not be surprising, as this test assesses patients in

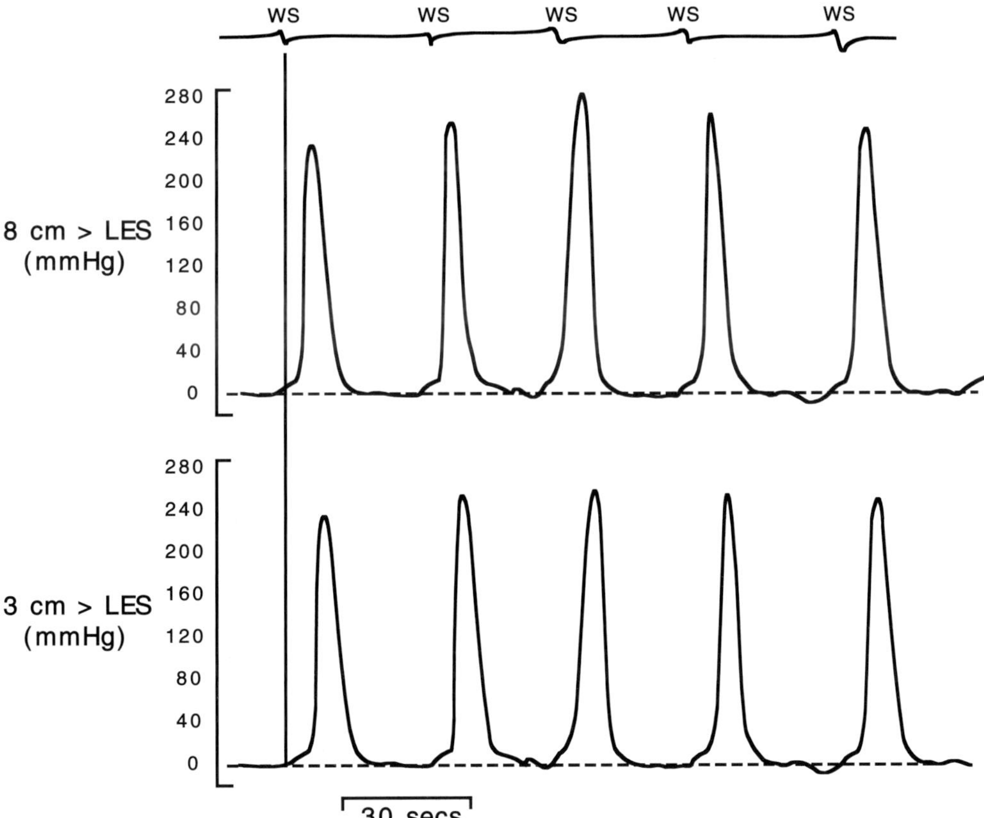

Fig 7–6. An esophageal manometry strip of the esophageal body, demonstrating high amplitude contractions (>180 mm Hg) in the distal esophagus, consistent with nutcracker esophagus.

a fasting, supine state, free of exogenous influences and with a rapid succession of wet and/or dry swallows.

Ambulatory 24-Hour Esophageal Manometry

Several groups have developed and reported their results in evaluating NCCP patients with prolonged ambulatory esophageal pressure monitors. This technology allows for 24-hour assessment of esophageal motility in the hope of capturing more spontaneous chest pain events while patients pursue their normal everyday activities. Hewson et al[40] evaluated 45 patients with NCCP who underwent baseline esophageal manometry with provocative testing and 24-hour esophageal pH and pressure monitoring. Standard esophageal manometry was abnormal in 20 (44%) patients. During ambulatory monitoring, all patients reported chest pain, but only in 26% of patients did symptoms occur during abnormal pH and/or motility abnormalities. The authors concluded that both pH and pressure monitoring are required to accurately define a relationship between chest pain and acid reflux or motility disorders.

Lacima et al[41] found that the addition of 24-hour esophageal manometry to the workup of NCCP patients produced only a minimal increase in the diagnostic yield. Abnormal esophageal motility was present in 42 (47%) patients as compared to 36 (40%) patients identified during stationary manometry tests. The lack of association between esophageal contractile abnormalities and chest pain[42-44] and the fact that the test is uncomfortable, requires a great deal of time to analyze, and is not widely available, makes

ambulatory 24-hour esophageal manometry not a useful diagnostic tool in clinical practice.[40]

Provocative Testing

In order to enhance the value of esophageal manometry in providing a definitive diagnosis, pharmacologic provocative agents have been used to elicit chest pain while monitoring changes in esophageal amplitude contractions

Edrophonium (Tensilon) Test

The edrophonium (Tensilon) test has been used pharmacologically to induce esophageal dysmotility and chest pain in patients with NCCP. Edrophonium is an anticholinesterase that increases cholinergic activity at muscarinic receptors.[45] The pharmacologic action of this short-acting drug is manifested within 30 to 60 seconds after injection and lasts an average of 10 minutes. The aim of the edrophonium test is to induce greater esophageal body amplitude contractions in the hope of provoking the patient's typical chest pain.[46] The test is performed by injection of either 80 mg/kg or 10 mg edrophonium IV, immediately followed by 5 to 10 swallows of 5 to 10 mL of water over a period of 5 to 10 minutes. The pain occurs during swallowing within 5 minutes after the administration of the drug and disappears as the drug is quickly metabolized.[47] Overall, the side effects are minimal, and the antidote atropine is rarely required. Side effects include increased salivation, nausea, vomiting, and abdominal cramps.

The sensitivity of the edrophonium test is relatively low. Studies have showed that the edrophonium test is positive in approximately 30% of patients with normal baseline esophageal manometry.[48,49] Consequently, the usage of the edrophonium test has declined in the last decade.

Ergonovine Stimulation Test

The ergonovine stimulation test has been demonstrated to induce augmentation of esophageal contractions and chest pain in patients with NCCP. Ergonovine is a sympathomimetic agent of the ergo-alkaloid group. The drug is reportedly as sensitive as edrophonium in the provocation of chest pain in NCCP patients, but the side effects are more common and could potentially be fatal (coronary artery spasm). Thus, ergonovine is rarely used today in clinical practice in the evaluation of NCCP.[47]

Pentagastrin Stimulation Test

Pentagastrin directly stimulates esophageal smooth muscle, especially in patients with primary esophageal dysmotility. Its sensitivity to inducing pain in patients with NCCP is low, and presently the drug is no longer used for NCCP provocative testing.[47]

Visceral Hyperalgesia

There are several tools that are used to assess the presence of visceral hyperalgesia, mostly within the realm of investigational studies. Intraesophageal balloon distension, either by barostat or by hand-held syringe, is the sole test that is used by some motility laboratories to provoke chest pain and to assess sensory perception thresholds.

Intraesophageal Balloon Distension Test

Intraesophageal balloon distension was reported to produce pain referred to the chest in human subjects about 50 years ago.[50] Fifteen years ago, the test was reintroduced as a provocative test in the evaluation of patients with NCCP.[51]

A small balloon is placed 10 cm above the LES and inflated at 1-mL increments to a total volume of 10 mL. Originally, inflations of the balloon were performed with a hand-held syringe. Subsequently, to ensure inflations at an accurate rate, a pump powered by compressed air was used. The introduction of the electronic barostat, a computer-driven volume-displacement device, provided simultaneous measurements of pressure for each balloon volume assessed. The pressure measurement helps to determine if the balloon remains within the esophagus. Increased balloon distensions result in increased esophageal contractions proximal to the balloon, in the attempt to propel the balloon into the stomach.[17] Migration of the balloon into the stomach could be detected by sudden drop in pressure measurements, despite increase in esophageal volumes (due to fundic receptive relaxation).

The basic principle of the barostat (Fig 7-7) is to maintain a constant pressure within the balloon or bag in the lumen despite esophageal muscular contractions and relaxations. To maintain a

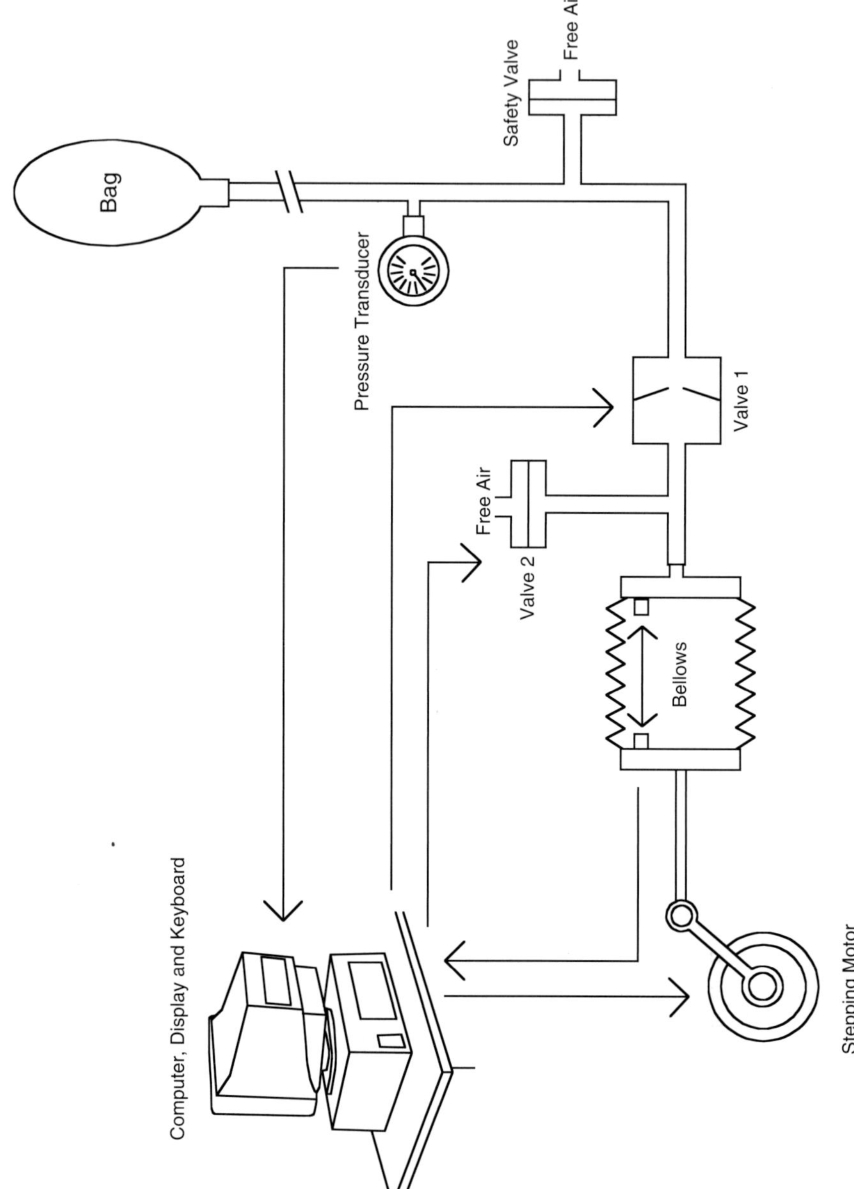

Fig 7-7. A schematic presentation of the electronic balloon distension device (the barostat).

constant pressure, the barostat aspirates air with muscular contractions and injects air with relaxations. At present, the use of a polyethylene bag is preferred over a latex balloon because it is infinitely compliant.[47]

Barish et al studied 30 patients with NCCP and 30 control subjects using an intraesophageal balloon distension protocol. The authors found that patients with NCCP were more likely to experience pain than normal controls (60 and 20%, respectively).[52] Moreover, patients with NCCP had chest pain at lower volumes of esophageal distension (8 mL vs 10 mL in normal volunteers).

Although patients with NCCP as a group have lower thresholds for pain than control subjects, the utility of this test in predicting the etiology of chest pain in NCCP patients has yet to be demonstrated in a prospective fashion. The balloon distension test is currently used primarily for research purposes to determine perception thresholds for pain.

Impedance Planimetry

This technique is primarily used to describe the biomechanical characteristics of the human esophagus.[53-55] The sensing system includes a thin latex balloon, which was used by some investigators to assess esophageal sensory thresholds. Balloon pressure was increased stepwise by 5 cm H_2O increments from 0 to determine sensory thresholds for pain in several studies.[54,56,57] After each inflation, the balloon was completely deflated for a rest period of 3 minutes. Balloon distensions were maintained each for 3 to 5 minutes. In this protocol, at each level of distension, the cross-sectional area

was measured and sensory response was determined using verbal descriptor. Grade 1 was considered a sensation of fullness, grade 2 was considered moderate discomfort, and grade 3 was considered severe pain. In validating this technique, the authors found that the threshold pressure required to induce a sensation of fullness varied between 20 and 50 cm H_2O.[54]

Summary

Evaluation for esophageal disorder in patients with NCCP should be undertaken after a cardiac cause has been excluded. Presence of alarm symptoms (Table 7–3) warrants initial evaluation with endoscopy or barium swallow if dysphagia is reported. However, if alarm symptoms are not reported by the patient, GERD should be excluded initially by using the PPI test or offering an empirical therapy with at least double-dose PPI over a period of 2 to 3 months. If the PPI test is negative or the patient did not respond to empirical therapy, a 24-hour esophageal pH monitoring on therapy should be considered. If the pH test is negative,

Table 7–3. Alarm Symptoms that, in the Presence of NCCP, Necessitate an Immediate Endoscopic Evaluation

- Dysphagia
- Odynophagia
- Anorexia
- Unintentional weight loss
- Fever
- Hematemesis/melena
- Repeated vomiting

esophageal manometry should be performed primarily to exclude achalasia. Provocative tests including balloon distension may be considered, but due to their limited sensitivity, potential side effects and lack of general availability are rarely performed. A diagnostic algorithm is proposed in Figure 7–8.

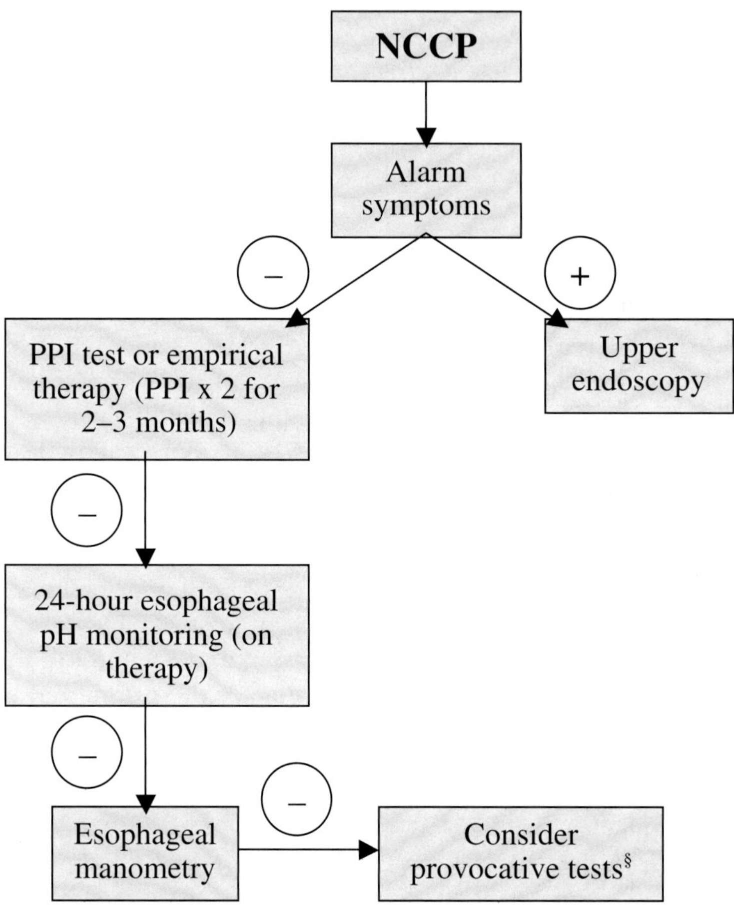

§ Acid perfusion test, edrophonium test, balloon distension test

Fig 7–8. Full proposed diagnostic algorithm for NCCP. (Repetition of previous performed negative tests was not shown to be helpful).[56]

References

1. Wong W-M, Risner-Adler S, Beeler J, et al. Noncardiac chest pain: the role of the cardiologist—a national survey. *J Clin Gastroenterol.* 2005;39(10):858-862.

2. Richter JE, Bradley LA, Castell DO. Esophageal chest pain: current controversies in pathogenesis, diagnosis, and therapy. *Ann Intern Med.* 1989;110(1):66-78.

3. Richter JE. Chest pain and gastroesophageal reflux disease. *J Clin Gastroenterol.* 2000;30 (3 suppl):S39-S41.

4. Shrestha S, Pasricha PJ. Update on noncardiac chest pain. *Dig Dis.* 2000;18(3):138-146.

5. Dekel R, Pearson T, Wendel C, DeGarmo P, Fennerty MB, Fass R. Assessment of oesophageal motor function in patients with dyspepsia or chest pain—the Clinical Outcomes Research Initiative experience. *Aliment Pharmacol Ther.* 2003;18(11-12):1083-1089.

6. Katz PO, Dalton CB, Richter JE, Wu WC, Castell DO. Esophageal testing of patients with noncardiac chest pain or dysphagia. Results of three years' experience with 1161 patients. *Ann Intern Med.* 1987;106(4):593-597.

7. Johnston BT, Troshinsky MB, Castell JA, Castell DO. Comparison of barium radiology with esophageal pH monitoring in the diagnosis of gastroesophageal reflux disease. *Am J Gastroenterol.* 1996;91(6):1181-1185.

8. Eslick GD, Fass R. Noncardiac chest pain: evaluation and treatment. *Gastroenterol Clin North Am.* 2003;32(2):531-552.

9. Fang J, Bjorkman D. A critical approach to noncardiac chest pain: pathophysiology, diagnosis, and treatment. *Am J Gastroenterol.* 2001;96(4):958-968.

10. Hsia PC, Maher KA, Lewis JH, Cattau EL, Jr., Fleischer DE, Benjamin SB. Utility of upper endoscopy in the evaluation of noncardiac chest pain. *Gastrointest Endosc.* 1991;37(1):22-26.

11. Frobert O, Funch-Jensen P, Jacobsen NO, Kruse A, Bagger JP. Upper endoscopy in patients with angina and normal coronary angiograms. *Endoscopy.* 1995;27(5):365-370.

12. Fass R, Fennerty MB, Ofman JJ, et al. The clinical and economic value of a short course of omeprazole in patients with noncardiac chest pain. *Gastroenterology.* 1998;115(1):42-49.

13. Bernstein LM, Baker LA. A clinical test for esophagitis. *Gastroenterology.* 1958;34(5):760-781.

14. Tack J, Janssens J. The esophagus and noncardiac chest pain. In: Castell DO, Richter JE, eds. *The Esophagus.* 4th ed. Philadelphia, Pa: Lippincott Williams & Wilkins; 2004:635-647.

15. Wu WC. Ancillary tests in the diagnosis of gastroesophageal reflux disease. *Gastroenterol Clin North Am.* 1990;19(3):671-682.

16. Pehlivanov N, Liu J, Mittal R. Abstract: Sustained esophageal contraction: a motor correlate of heartburn symptom. *Gastroenterology.* 1999;116(4):A1062, G4613.

17. Fass R, Naliboff B, Higa L, et al. Differential effect of long-term esophageal acid exposure on mechanosensitivity and chemosensitivity in humans. *Gastroenterology.* 1998;115(6):1363-1373.

18. Gracely RH, McGrath P, Dubner R. Ratio scales of sensory and affective verbal pain descriptors. *Pain.* 1978;5:5-18.

19. Hewson EG, Sinclair JW, Dalton CB, Richter JE. Twenty-four-hour esophageal pH monitoring: the most useful test for evaluating noncardiac chest pain. *Am J Med.* 1991;90(5):576-583.

20. Dekel R, Martinez-Hawthorne SD, Guillen RJ, Fass R. Evaluation of symptom index in identifying gastroesophageal reflux disease-related noncardiac chest pain. *J Clin Gastroenterol.* 2004;38(1):24-29.

21. Paterson WG. Canadian Association of Gastroenterology Practice Guidelines: management of noncardiac chest pain. *Can J Gastroenterol.* 1998;12(6):401-407.

22. Faybush EM, Fass R. Gastroesophageal reflux disease in noncardiac chest pain. *Gastroenterol Clin North Am.* 2004; 33(1):41-54.

23. Pandolfino JE, Richter JE, Ourts T, Guardino JM, Chapman J, Karhrilas PJ. Ambulatory esophageal pH monitoring using a wireless system. *Am J Gastroenterol.* 2003;98(4):740-749.

24. Prakash C, Clouse R. Wireless pH monitoring in patients with non-cardiac chest pain. *Am J Gastroenterol.* 2006;101: 446-452.

25. Fass R. Unexplained chest pain. *Curr Opin Gastroenterol.* 2002;18:464-470.

26. Young MF, Sanowski RA, Talbert GA, et al. [abstract]: Omeprazole administration as a test for gastroesophageal reflux. *Gastroenterology.* 1992;102:192.

27. Squillace SJ, Young MF, Sanowski RA. Single dose omeprazole as a test for noncardiac chest pain [abstract]. *Gastroenterology.* 1993;107:A197.

28. Fass R, Pulliam G, Hayden CW. Patients with non-cardiac chest pain (NCCP) receiving an empirical trial of high dose lansoprazole, demonstrate early symptom response—a double blind, placebo-controlled trial (abstract). *Gastroenterology.* 2001;122:A580, W1175.

29. Fass R, Fullerton H, Hayden CW, Garewal HS. Patients with noncardiac chest pain (NCCP) receiving an empirical trial of high dose rabeprazole, demonstrate early symptom response—a double blind, placebo-controlled trial (abstract). *Gastroenterology.* 2002;122:A580, W1175.

30. Xia HH, Lai KC, Lam SK, et al. Symptomatic response to lansoprazole predicts abnormal acid reflux in endoscopy-negative patients with non-cardiac chest pain. *Aliment Pharmacol Ther.* 2003; 17:369-377.

31. Pandak WM, Arezo S, Everett S, et al. Short course of omeprazole: A better first diagnostic approach to noncardiac chest pain than endoscopy, manometry, or 24-hour esophageal pH monitoring. *J Clin Gastroenterol.* 2002;35:307-314.

32. Ofman JJ, Gralnek IM, Udani J, Fennerty MB, Fass R. The cost-effectiveness of the omeprazole test in patients with noncardiac chest pain. *Am J Med.* 1999;107(3): 219-227.

33. Carlsson R, Galmiche JP, Dent J, Lundell L, Frison L. Prognostic factors influencing relapse of oesophagitis during maintenance therapy with antisecretory drugs: a meta-analysis of long-term omeprazole trials. *Aliment Pharmacol Ther.* 1997; 11(3):473-482.

34. Azpiroz F, Dapoigny M, Pace F, et al. Non-gastrointestinal disorders in the irritable bowel syndrome. *Digestion.* 2000;62(1): 66-72.

35. Ali M, Lacy B. Esophaeal manometry and pH monitoring: gastroenterologists' adherence to published guidelines. *J Clin Gastroenterol.* 2005;39(7):584-590.

36. Clouse RE, Lustman PJ, Eckert TC, Ferney DM, Griffith LS. Low-dose trazodone for symptomatic patients with esophageal contraction abnormalities. A double-blind, placebo-controlled trial. *Gastroenterology.* 1987;92(4):1027-1036.

37. Fass R, Winters GF. Primary care focus: evaluation of the patient with NCCP—Is GERD or an esophageal motility disorder the cause? *Medscape Gastroenterol.* 2001;3(6):1-15.

38. Knippig C, Fass R, P M. Tests for the evaluation of functional gastrointestinal disorders. *Dig Dis.* 2001;19(3):232-239.

39. DiMarino AJ, Jr., Allen ML, Lynn RB, Zamani S. Clinical value of esophageal motility testing. *Dig Dis.* 1998;16(4): 198-204.

40. Hewson EG, Dalton CB, Richter JE. Comparison of esophageal manometry, provocative testing, and ambulatory monitoring in patients with unexplained chest pain. *Dig Dis Sci.* 1990;35(3):302-309.

41. Lacima G, Grande L, Pera M, Francino A, Ros E. Utility of ambulatory 24-hour esophageal pH and motility monitoring in noncardiac chest pain: report of 90 patients and review of the literature. *Dig Dis Sci.* 2003;48(5):952-961.

42. Peters L, Mass L, Petty D, et al. Spontaneous noncardiac chest pain. Evaluation by 24-hour ambulatory esophageal motility and pH monitoring. *Gastroenterology.* 1988;94(4):878-886.

43. Breumelhof R, Nadorp JH, Akkermans LM, Smout AJ. Analysis of 24-hour esophageal pressure and pH data in unselected patients with noncardiac chest pain. *Gastroenterology.* 1990;99(5):1257-1264.

44. Cameron R, Barclay M, Dobbs B. Ambulatory oesophageal manometry and pH monitoring for investigation of chest pain: a New Zealand experience. *N Z Med J.* 2006;119(1230):U1877.

45. London RL, Ouyang A, Snape WJJ, et al. Provocation of esophageal pain by ergonovine or edrophonium. *Gastroenterology.* 1981;81:10-14.

46. Nostrant TT. Provocation testing in noncardiac chest pain. *Am J Med.* 1992; 92(5A):56S-64S.

47. Fass R. Provocative Tests for Pain of Esophageal Origin. In: Castell DO, Richter JE, eds. *The Esophagus.* 4th ed. Philadelphia, Pa: Lippincott Williams & Wilkins; 2004:165-183.

48. Lee C, Reynolds J, Ouyang A, Baker L, Cohen S. Esophageal chest pain. Value of high-dose provocative testing with edrophonium chloride in patients with normal esophageal manometries. *Dig Dis Sci.* 1987;32(7):682-688.

49. Richter JE, Hackshaw BT, Wu WC, Castell DO. Edrophonium: a useful provocative test for esophageal chest pain. *Ann Intern Med.* 1985;103(1):14-21.

50. Kramer P, Hollander W. Comparison of experimental esophageal pain with clinical pain of angina pectoris and esophageal disease. *Gastroenterology.* 1955; 29(5):719-743.

51. Richter JE, Barish CF, Castell DO. Abnormal sensory perception in patients with esophageal chest pain. *Gastroenterology.* 1986;91(4):845-852.

52. Barish CF, Castell DO, Richter JE. Graded esophageal balloon distention. A new provocative test for noncardiac chest pain. *Dig Dis Sci.* 1986;31(12):1292-1298.

53. Silny J, Knigge KP, Fass J, et al. Verification of the intraluminal multiple electrical impedance measurement for the recording of gastrointestinal motility. *J Gastrointest Motil.* 1993;5:107-122.

54. Rao SSC, Hayek B, Summers RW. Impedance planimetry: an integrated approach for assessing sensory, active, and passive biomechanical properties of the human esophagus. *Am J Gastroenterol.* 1995; 90(3):431-438.

55. Orvar KB, Gregersen H, Christensen J. Biomechanical characteristics of the human esophagus. *Dig Dis Sci.* 1993; 38(2):197-205.

56. Randich A. Visceral nerve stimulation and pain modulation. In: Josh LR, ed. *Physiology of the Gastrointestinal Tract.* 3rd ed. New York, NY: Oxford University; 1993:126-139.

57. Rao SSC, Hayek B, Summers RW. Functional chest pain of esophageal origin: hyperalgesia or motor dysfunction. *Am J Gastroenterol.* 2001;96(9):2584-2589.

CHAPTER 8

The Proton-Pump Inhibitor (PPI) Therapeutic Trial

Wai-Man Wong
Ronnie Fass

Introduction

The diagnostic tests currently available for GERD include barium esophagram, upper endoscopy, esophageal manometry, and ambulatory 24-hour esophageal pH monitoring. Barium esophagram is considered an inappropriate initial test for the evaluation of patients with heartburn.[1] Generally, it has a very low sensitivity and specificity for the diagnosis of GERD although the sensitivity improves somewhat in higher grades of erosive esophagitis. Moreover, barium reflux during an esophagram is of questionable significance and can be demonstrated in up to 20% of healthy subjects.[2] Presently, barium esophagram should be considered primarily in patients with GERD that present with dysphagia.

The sensitivity of upper endoscopy in patients with typical GERD symptoms is approximately 30 to 50%, mainly because most patients with GERD (50 to 70%) lack any evidence of esophageal mucosal injury.[1,3] However, upper endoscopy is the gold standard for diagnosing esophageal mucosal injury due to GERD (erosive esophagitis, ulceration, peptic stricture, and Barrett's esophagus). Furthermore, upper endoscopy allows the assessment of the degree of mucosal involvement (erosive esophagitis grading) and the presence of dysplasia in Barrett's esophagus. It appears that there is little value for histopathologic examination of normal appearing esophageal mucosa in patients with normal endoscopy to either confirm or exclude GERD.

Esophageal manometry has no role in the diagnosis of GERD because most patients lack any significant esophageal manometric changes. The study is indicated primarily in patients with GERD who are candidates for antireflux surgery to exclude achalasia or ineffective peristalsis (<30 mm Hg).

For a long time, ambulatory 24-hour esophageal pH monitoring has been regarded as the gold standard for diagnosing GERD. Reported sensitivity has ranged from 79 to 96% and specificity from 85 to 100%.[4-6] However, recent studies have found that 24-hour esophageal pH monitoring is normal in up to 25% of the patients with erosive esophagitis and 50% of the patients with nonerosive reflux disease.[7-9]

In addition to the limited sensitivity of the above aforementioned diagnostic tests for GERD, these tests are invasive, costly, and may not be readily available to many community-based physicians.

The Proton-Pump Inhibitor Therapeutic Trial (PPI Test)

The PPI therapeutic trial or the PPI test is defined as a short course of high-dose PPI for diagnosing GERD. This is a simple and noninvasive diagnostic tool for GERD. It is readily available and at the disposal of every primary care physician. Additionally, it increases the role of primary care physicians in evaluating and treating patients with different manifestations of GERD. It also offers significant cost savings when compared to the other diagnostic tests for GERD.

Empirical therapy with PPIs (usually 2–3 months of treatment) has often been used by physicians as the initial treatment of patients with typical or atypical manifestations of GERD. However, it is both impractical and costly for patients to complete several months or longer of acid suppression therapy before determining whether the medication is of benefit or not.[7]

The doses used in PPI therapeutic trials have ranged from 40 mg to 80 mg daily for omeprazole, 30 mg to 60 mg daily for lansoprazole, and 40 mg daily for rabeprazole, over duration of treatment of 1 to 28 days, in patients with symptoms suggestive of GERD or noncardiac chest pain (NCCP) (Tables 8–1 and 8–2).[7,8,10-20] In patients with laryngeal manifestations of GERD, the doses ranged from 40 mg to 80 mg omeprazole daily and the duration of treatment from 1 to 4 weeks.[21-24] By far, the most commonly used PPI in most of the therapeutic trials is omeprazole, which has led to the term the "omeprazole test."[7,8,10-17,21-23] However, studies using other PPIs demonstrated that they are equally efficacious as therapeutic trial.[18-20]

An important factor in determining the sensitivity of a therapeutic trial is the definition of a positive test. In most studies, a symptom score cutoff was used: if the symptom assessment score for heartburn, chest pain, or other symptoms improved by more than 50 to 75% (depending on the study) relative to baseline, the test was considered positive. As with any diagnostic test, the optimal cutoff is critical in defining test accuracy.[25] The symptom score cutoff values that were used among studies that evaluated therapeutic trials for GERD were chosen arbitrarily. Rarely, studies calculated the Receiver Operator Curve (ROC) by varying the percentage reduction in the symptom tested to ascertain the optimal value for detecting patients with GERD.[7,12,25] This cutoff point provides the greatest sensitivity, specificity, positive predictive value, and accuracy of the therapeutic trial tested.

As with any other test, the sensitivity of a therapeutic trial depends on the

Table 8–1. Proton-Pump Inhibitor Empirical Trials in GERD

First Author	Reference	Dosing Schedule	No. of Patients	% Symptom Improvement	Sensitivity (%)	Specificity (%)
Schindlbeck	10	Omeprazole 40 mg/day × 7 days Omeprazole 40 mg twice daily × 7 days	11	75	27	*NA
Schenk	8	Omeprazole 40 mg/day × 14 days	85	At least 2 grades improvement in symptom score	68	63
Johnsson	11	Omeprazole 20 mg twice daily × 7 days	160	At least 1 grade improvement in symptom score	75	55
Fass	12	Omeprazole (40 mg in the morning and 20 mg in the evening) for 7 days	42	50	80	57
Juul-Hansen	14	Lansoprazole 60 mg/day × 5 days	64	Reduction in antacid consumption = 75%	85	73
Bate	13	Omeprazole 40 mg/day × 14 days	90	Improvement in heartburn symptoms by 2 grades	89	35

Table 8–2. Proton-Pump Inhibitor Therapeutic Trials in NCCP

First Author	Reference	Dosing Schedule	No. of Patients	Symptom Improvement- (%)	Sensitivity (%)	Specificity (%)
Young	16	Omeprazole 80 mg/day × 1 day	30	75	90	80
Squillace	15	Omeprazole 80 mg/day × 1 day	17	50	69	75
Xia	18	Lansoprazole 30 mg/day × 4 weeks	68	50	92	67
Pandak	17	Omeprazole 40 mg twice daily × 2 weeks	37	50	90	67
Fass	7	Omeprazole (40 mg in the morning and 20 mg in the evening) for 7 days	37	50	78	86
Fass	19	Lansoprazole (60 mg in the morning and 30 mg in the evening) for 7 days	40	50	78	82
Fass	20	Rabeprazole (20 mg in the morning and 20 mg in the evening) for 7 days	20	50	83	75

prevalence of the disease in the patient population that is evaluated. Obviously, the therapeutic trial has minimal utility in patients with erosive esophagitis, in whom acid reflux is almost always the underlying cause. However, as the likelihood of a particular syndrome being attributable to reflux decreases, the potential value of a therapeutic trial increases.

The diagnostic accuracy of the PPI therapeutic trial is limited by the lack of a gold standard for the diagnosis of GERD.

In the absence of a gold standard, studies evaluating the PPI therapeutic trials have used a combination of upper endoscopy and ambulatory 24-hour esophageal pH monitoring as the closest one can get to a gold standard. Factors that may determine the sensitivity of the PPI therapeutic trial are listed in Table 8–3.

Only one study attempted to compare the accuracy of the PPI therapeutic trial (omeprazole test) versus 24-hour esophageal pH monitoring in diagnosing GERD.[26] The study used the presence of erosive esophagitis as indicative of GERD in patients who are not on ASA or NSAIDs. Thirty-five patients were included, and they underwent both pH testing and the PPI therapeutic trial (omeprazole 40 mg in the morning and 20 mg in the evening). The PPI therapeutic trial was significantly more sensitive than total acid contact time during pH testing (83% vs 60%, p <0.03). The sensitivity of the pH test increased to 80% only after adding patients with positive symptom index, and patients with abnormal acid contact time in the supine and erect positions despite normal total acid contact time. The authors concluded that the PPI therapeutic trial was at least as sensitive as

Table 8–3. Factors that Determine the Sensitivity of a Proton-Pump Inhibitor Therapeutic Trial

Type of antireflux medication used

Dosage

Treatment duration

Definition of a positive test (symptom score cutoff, change in symptom grading, receiver operating characteristics curve analysis)

GERD-related symptom evaluated

ambulatory 24-hour esophageal pH monitoring in diagnosing GERD in patients with documented erosive esophagitis.

PPI Therapeutic Trial in GERD

Several studies have assessed the usefulness of the PPI therapeutic trial in patients with typical symptoms (heartburn and/or acid regurgitation) of GERD. Patients recruited into these studies include patients with nonerosive reflux disease (normal upper endoscopy but abnormal 24-hour esophageal pH monitoring) [8,10-14] or symptomatic GERD patients (not limited to specific esophageal findings).[8,11-13] In many of these studies, response to the PPI therapeutic trial was indicative of GERD as the underlying cause of symptoms. All these studies assessed the ability of the PPI therapeutic trial to diagnose patients with abnormal upper endoscopy and/or abnormal 24-hour esophageal pH monitoring. The dosages of PPIs used ranged from 40 mg to 80 mg daily for omeprazole [8,10-13] and 60 mg daily for lansoprazole.[14] Most studies determined that 7 days of treatment was sufficient to provide maximum sensitivity.[10-12] Reported sensitivity of the PPI therapeutic trial ranged from 27 to 89% and specificity from 35 to 73%.[8,10-14] Due to different methodologies as well as patient populations, comparison between these studies is difficult. However, Schindlbeck et al have shown that omeprazole 40 mg daily for 7 days provided a sensitivity of 27% only, which increased to 83% if the dose was increased to 40 mg twice daily.[10] Fass et al have demonstrated that a lower dose of omeprazole 60 mg daily (40 mg in the morning and 20 mg in the evening) for 7 days provided equally satisfactory sensitivity of 80%.[12] In the latter study, the omeprazole test was considered positive when the heartburn intensity score improved by at least 50% on treatment. However, if the cutoff for a positive test was at least 75% improvement in symptom response, the sensitivity would have increased to 86% with a positive predictive value of 91% and an accuracy of 81%.[12]

Assessment of the diagnostic accuracy of the PPI therapeutic trial in symptomatic GERD patients or those with nonerosive reflux disease is limited by the lack of a gold standard for GERD. Additionally, the specificity of the PPI therapeutic trial in GERD was found to be relatively low due to positive response to the treatment, albeit limited, by those patients with normal upper endoscopy and normal 24-hour esophageal pH monitoring. This group of patients has been defined as having functional heartburn according to Rome III criteria for functional esophageal disorders.[27] A subset of these patients may still respond to the PPI therapeutic trial, because their underlying mechanism for heartburn is hypersensitivity to gastroesophageal reflux.[8,12,14] These patients termed "the hypersensitive esophagus" appear to be sensitive to acid reflux within the physiological range (normal).[28] Patients with the hypersensitive esophagus may respond to PPI therapy although more than once a day PPI is commonly needed.[29]

Numans et al[30] assessed the value of the PPI test in diagnosing GERD in patients with atypical GERD symptoms. They concluded that successful short-term treatment with a PPI in patients suspected of having GERD does not confidently establish the diagnosis when GERD is defined by currently accepted reference standards. However, when validating a new diagnostic tool, comparison to the gold standard is necessary. Because there is no diagnostic gold standard for GERD, combination of an upper endoscopy and 24-hour esophageal pH monitoring has been considered as the closest one can get to a gold standard. When both of these tests are used, then the functional heartburn group is expected to be the excluded group. Approximately 50% of the functional heartburn patients demonstrate response to standard dose PPI therapy.[31] Moreover, higher doses of PPI further increase the response rate of functional heartburn patients, primarily those with hypersensitive esophagus.[29] These findings explain the low specificity that the PPI tests have achieved in patients with classic GERD symptoms. Alternatively, the PPI test may be highly valuable in GERD, because it can detect those patients with functional heartburn who are responsive to antireflux therapy.

In summary, the PPI therapeutic trial in patients with typical GERD symptoms allows physicians to have a fast and fairly accurate tool for diagnosing GERD. Patients who respond to the PPI therapeutic trial may be stepped down to a lower dose of PPI or even to H_2 receptor antagonist (H_2RA). However, none of the studies thus far have evaluated if a positive response to the PPI therapeutic trial is predictive of long-term response to antireflux treatment.

PPI Therapeutic Trial in Noncardiac Chest Pain

Noncardiac chest pain (NCCP) is defined as recurrent episodes of retrosternal pain in patients with no cardiac abnormality.[32,33] It has been estimated that the prevalence of NCCP is 23% in a large population-based study.[34] Up to 30% of the coronary angiograms performed annually for patients with chest pain are normal. Considering that at least 600,000 coronary angiograms are performed each year in the United States for chest pain of recent onset, then NCCP is diagnosed in nearly 180,000 patients annually.[35] However, this is largely an underestimate of the extent of the problem because in many patients diagnosed with NCCP, cardiac angiogram is deemed unnecessary.

GERD is the cause of symptoms in up to 60% of patients with NCCP.[36-38] In addition, antireflux treatment results in marked improvement in symptoms of these patients. The diagnostic tools that have been commonly used for the evaluation of patients with NCCP, after a normal cardiac investigation, were upper endoscopy, 24-hour esophageal pH monitoring, esophageal manometry, and provocative testing (the acid perfusion test, Tensilon test, and balloon distension test).[32,33] However, these tests are invasive, expensive, and not readily available for many physicians. In contrast, the PPI therapeutic trial is a simple, noninvasive, and readily available method for diagnosing patients with GERD-related NCCP.

The sensitivity of the PPI therapeutic trial for GERD-related NCCP ranged from 69 to 95% and the specificity from 67 to 86% (see Table 8–2).[7,15-20] The dosages of PPIs used ranged from 60 mg to 80 mg daily for omeprazole;[7,15-17] 30 mg to 90 mg for lansoprazole;[18,19] and 40 mg for rabeprazole.[20] The trial duration ranged from 1 to 28 days.[7,15-20]

In two early studies, a single dose of 80 mg omeprazole was tested resulting in variable sensitivity (69 to 90%).[15,16] However, in these studies patients were crossed over to the opposite arm after a

washout period of 2 to 5 days, which may be too short and result in carryover effect. Subsequently, in a double-blind, placebo-controlled trial, 37 patients with NCCP were randomized to either placebo or high-dose omeprazole (40 mg in the morning and 20 mg in the evening) for 7 days.[7] After a washout period and repeated baseline symptom assessment, patients crossed over to the opposite arm. The PPI therapeutic trial was considered positive if the chest pain improved by at least 50% after treatment. The combination of upper endoscopy and 24-hour esophageal pH monitoring was used as the gold standard. Sixty-two percent (23/37) of the patients had evidence of GERD: seven had abnormal esophageal acid exposure by pH testing only, eight had erosive esophagitis only, and eight had both. Of the GERD-positive group, 78.3% had a positive PPI therapeutic trial, and 22.7% had a positive placebo response. In contrast, of the GERD-negative group, 14.2% had a positive PPI therapeutic trial, and 7.1% had a positive placebo response. Thus, the calculated sensitivity was 78.3%, specificity 85.7%, and the positive predictive value was 90%.[7] When different reductions in chest pain were evaluated as previously mentioned, the greater accuracy of predicting GERD-related NCCP was obtained with 65% symptom reduction, producing a sensitivity of 85.7% and specificity of 90.9%.[7] Using similar design, other investigators confirmed the usefulness of the PPI therapeutic trial for diagnosing GERD-related NCCP.[17,18] Furthermore, in subsequent studies, Fass et al demonstrated that therapeutic trials with PPIs other than omeprazole achieve similar efficacy for the diagnosis of GERD-related NCCP.[19,20] A recent study in the Chinese population showed that PPI therapeutic trial, using lansoprazole 30 mg daily for a period of 4 weeks, was useful diagnosing endoscopy-negative GERD-related NCCP.[18]

In a recent meta-analysis of randomized, controlled trials (parallel group and crossover design), the authors evaluated the pooled risk ratio for continued chest pain after PPI therapy, overall number needed to treat, and pool sensitivity, specificity, and diagnostic odds ratio for the PPI test versus reference standards.[39]

Eight studies were included in the PPI efficacy analysis. The pooled risk ratio for continued chest pain after PPI therapy was 0.54 (95% confidence interval [CI], 0.41-0.71). The overall number needed to treat was 3 (95% CI, 2-4). The pooled sensitivity, specificity, and diagnostic odds ratio for the PPI test versus 24-hour pH monitoring and upper endoscopy were 80%, 73%, and 13.83 (95% CI, 5.48-34.91), respectively. All studies were small, and there was evidence of publication bias or other small study effects. The authors concluded that PPI therapy reduces symptoms in NCCP and may be useful as a diagnostic test in identifying abnormal esophageal acid reflux. However, in this meta-analysis, the authors included a potpourri of diagnostic and therapeutic trials with a PPI in patients with NCCP. Many of these trials have little in common and often used different clinical endpoints. Of the 8 studies included in the PPI efficacy analysis, 2 (25%) were published only in an abstract form.[15,20] Additionally, one study[40] focused on the value of the ph testing-derived parameter—the symptom index in patients with NCCP. The usage of an open-label PPI test in these patients was a secondary endpoint. Another study[18] was done exclusively in Chinese patients with nonerosive reflux disease-related NCCP. Furthermore, the latter study

included a standard dose PPI given during a period of 1 month. One study[41] was an open-label, empirical therapy in patients with NCCP, using omeprazole 40 mg in the evening during a period of 6 weeks. The studies differ significantly from each other in many clinical aspects, which adversely affected the quality of the meta-analysis.

Wang et al have also performed a meta-analysis of the PPI test in patients with NCCP.[42] Unlike the previous meta-analysis, the authors found only 6 studies that met inclusion criteria. The overall sensitivity and specificity of a PPI test were 80% (95% CI, 71-87%) and 74% (95% CI, 12-29%), and 77% (95% CI, 62-87%), respectively, in the placebo group. The PPI test showed significant higher discriminative power, with a summary diagnostic odds ratio of 19.35 (95% CI, 8.54-43.84) compared to 0.61 (95% CI, 0.20-1.86) in the placebo group. Thus, the authors concluded that the use of PPI treatment as a diagnostic test for detecting GERD in patients with NCCP has an acceptable sensitivity and specificity and could be used as an initial approach by primary care physicians to detect GERD in selected patients with NCCP.

When using the PPI therapeutic trial, there was a significant correlation between the extent of esophageal acid exposure in the distal esophagus as determined by ambulatory 24-hour esophageal pH monitoring and the change in symptom intensity score after treatment, suggesting that the higher the esophageal acid exposure, the greater the response to the PPI therapeutic trial in patients with GERD-related NCCP.[43]

Economic analysis showed that the PPI therapeutic trial for GERD-related NCCP is a cost-saving approach primarily due to significant reduction in the usage of various costly, invasive diagnostic tests.[7]

PPI Therapeutic Trial for Extraesophageal Manifestations of GERD

The PPI therapeutic trial has increasingly become important in patients with extraesophageal manifestation of GERD. Although the association between GERD and various oropharyngeal, laryngeal, and pulmonary disorders has been documented, the extent of causality remains unknown.[21,44-46] Furthermore, assessment of the role of the PPI therapeutic trial in extraesophageal manifestations of GERD is also hampered by the lack of a gold standard for diagnosing GERD. However, response to the PPI therapeutic trial is indicative for a causal relationship between these disorders and GERD and thus may obviate the need for a battery of invasive diagnostic tests.

The required dosage and duration of the PPI therapeutic trial in patients with suspected extraesophageal manifestations of GERD are yet to be determined. Dosages and durations used in GERD and NCCP may well be insufficient. Therapeutic studies have shown that patients with extraesophageal manifestations of GERD may require higher doses of PPI and longer duration of treatment (up to 6 months) to obtain a satisfactory response.[36,47-50]

Thus far, only a few studies have examined the utility of the PPI therapeutic trial in patients with extraesophageal manifestations of GERD. In a pilot study of 10 patients with laryngeal symptoms, omeprazole 20 mg twice daily was prescribed for 1 month.[21] The PPI therapeutic trial had a sensitivity of 62.5%. However, the study was open label, and a placebo group was not included. Three studies assessed the usefulness of the PPI therapeutic trial in patients with chronic cough. In the first study, omeprazole 20 mg was administered 3 times daily over a period of 7 days, and response was assessed by improvement in cough symptom score. The reported sensitivity of the PPI therapeutic trial was 81%, and specificity was 92%.[23] In the second study, 23 patients with chronic cough received omeprazole 40 mg twice daily for 12 weeks. The authors found that those who responded to the PPI therapeutic trial did so within 5 to 14 days.[22] However, the sensitivity of the PPI therapeutic trial was only 35% in this study. In the third study, the author used a crossover design to study the effect of omeprazole 40 mg daily versus placebo in 21 patients with GERD-related chronic cough over a period of 8 weeks.[24] Interpretation of the results of this study are limited by the presence of a significant carryover effect (the effect achieved from the omeprazole persisted into the placebo treatment phase). In this study, cough symptoms improved significantly during omeprazole treatment in 57% of the patients who initially received placebo and subsequently crossed over to the omeprazole arm.

Cost-Effectiveness

In a decision analysis model, the potential economic impact of an initial noninvasive diagnostic strategy—the PPI therapeutic trial—was compared to the traditional invasive diagnostic strategy in patients with symptoms suggestive of GERD.[12] This model estimated financial and clinical outcome over a 1-year period. The decision analysis is based on the assumption that the results of the PPI therapeutic trial are believed, and that the clinicians treat for GERD if the trial is positive and pursue an alternative diagnosis if the trial is negative. The results of this economic analysis demonstrated that the PPI therapeutic trial saves $347 per average patient with symptoms suggestive of GERD undergoing diagnostic evaluation. The cost savings are due to 64% reduction in the number of upper endoscopies and 53% reduction in utilization of pH tests. These findings were confirmed by a subsequent study.[13]

Similarly, in patients with NCCP, the PPI therapeutic trial was evaluated using a cost-minimization analysis.[7] The PPI therapeutic trial was found to save $573 per average patient with NCCP undergoing diagnostic evaluation. The trial was associated with an 81% reduction in the number of upper endoscopies and 79% reduction in the number of ambulatory 24-hour esophageal pH tests. This significant reduction is due to the high positive predictive value of the PPI therapeutic trial for patients with GERD-related NCCP.

When a decision-analytic model utilizing Bayesian analysis was developed to compare the costs and outcomes of alternative diagnostic strategies for NCCP, noninvasive strategies utilizing the PPI therapeutic trial as the initial step resulted in significant cost savings as compared to invasive strategies. These cost savings were a direct result of a significant reduction in the utilization of invasive diagnostic tests that are of unproven utility in the diagnosis and subsequent management of patients with NCCP.[37]

A decision analysis in patients with GERD calculated the clinical and economic outcomes of competing management strategies.[38] The traditional strategy incorporated sequential therapeutic trials with more intensive therapy ("step-up" approach) followed by sequential invasive diagnostic testing of nonresponders. The PPI therapeutic trial (test) strategy included an initial PPI test (7 days of omeprazole 40 mg AM and 20 mg PM daily) followed by less intensive therapeutic trials in those testing positive ("step-down" approach) with sequential invasive diagnostic testing as needed.

The average cost per patient was $1,045 for the traditional step-up management strategy, compared to $1,172 for the "PPI test" and step-down strategy. The percentage of patients who were symptom free at 1 year was 50% for the traditional management strategy compared to 75% for the "PPI test" strategy. The incremental cost-effectiveness ratio for the "PPI therapeutic trial" strategy is $510 per additional symptomatic cure over 1 year, and between $2,822 to $10,160 per quality-adjusted life years gained.

Empirical Therapy with PPIs

Empirical therapy with a PPI is commonly used in clinical practice. Diagnosis of GERD may be based on classic symptoms, such as heartburn and acid regurgitation, and subsequently patients are treated empirically with a PPI for the acute (2–3 months) and maintenance periods.[51] A different clinical approach may use the response to an empirical therapy with a PPI as a confirmation for the diagnosis of GERD. The latter approach has been expanded into the area of atypical and extraesophageal manifestations of GERD. For example, patients that present with NCCP receive an empirical therapy with a PPI twice daily for a period of 2 months.[52] Instead of initiating a diagnostic workup with the PPI therapeutic trial or other available tests, the physician elects to use the response to the empirical therapy as the determining factor if diagnostic evaluation is needed or patients can safely continue into the maintenance phase of their treatment. In extraesophageal manifestations of GERD, a similar approach as in NCCP has been adopted, although the duration of the empirical therapy may be extended to 6 months.[53]

Summary

The use of the PPI therapeutic trial in patients with symptoms suggestive of GERD and NCCP provides simplicity, diagnostic accuracy, and cost savings that patients and physicians are seeking when establishing the diagnosis of GERD. The therapeutic trial is easily performed, relatively inexpensive, and at the disposal of most primary care physicians. In addition, this powerful diagnostic tool may increase the role of community-based physicians in evaluating and subsequently treating patients with typical symptoms suggestive of GERD and NCCP. Furthermore, the usage of the PPI therapeutic trial as the initial diagnostic step may result in significant cost savings to health plans and third-party payers. Results of initial studies assessing the effectiveness of the therapeutic trial in patients with extraesophageal manifestations of GERD are promising, but further research is needed.

The clinical need for the PPI therapeutic trial increases as the true prevalence of GERD in esophageal (erosive esophagitis, nonerosive reflux disease, and NCCP) and extraesophageal manifestations (ENT, asthma, and miscellaneous) decreases (Fig 8-1).[25] In addition, it

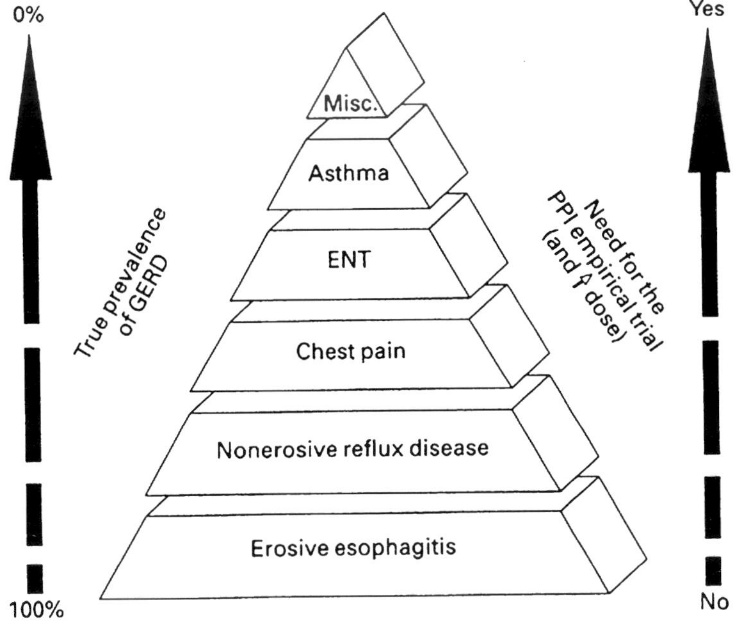

Fig 8–1. The PPI therapeutic pyramid. As the true prevalence of GERD decreases in the various esophageal and extraesophageal manifestations of GERD, then the need for the PPI therapeutic trial increases as well as the required dosage. (Adapted from Fass R. *Dig Dis*. 2000;18:20–26.)

appears that the need for increased dose of PPI in the therapeutic trial is inversely related to the true prevalence of GERD in the esophageal manifestations as represented in the "pyramid" of the disease.

In summary, the PPI therapeutic trial is a valuable diagnostic tool for the diag- nosis of the different phenotypic presentations of GERD and should be incorporated into the arsenal of diagnostic tools of primary care physicians and subspecialists. A diagnostic algorithm is proposed in Figure 8–2.

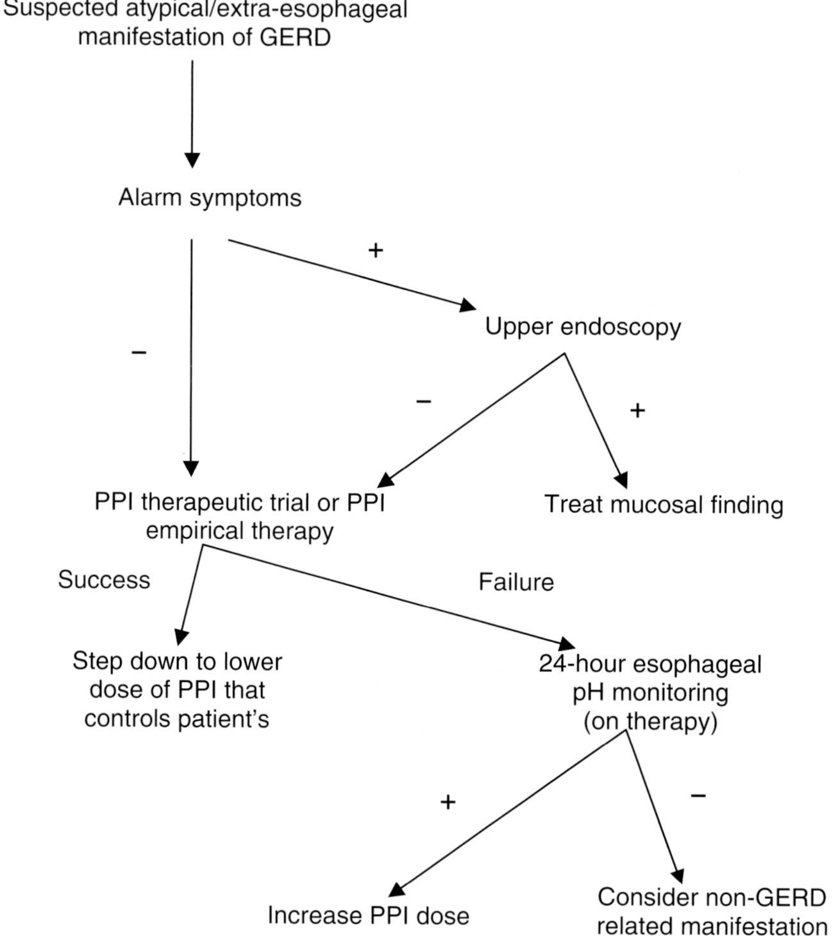

Fig 8–2. A therapeutic algorithm for typical and atypical/extraesophageal manifestations of GERD.

References

1. Joseph S, Hirano I. Gastroesophageal reflux disease: diagnosis. In: Fass R, ed. *GERD/Dyspepsia: Hot Topics*. Philadelphia, Pa: Hanley & Belfus, Inc; 2004: 41–54.
2. Wu W. Ancillary tests in the diagnosis of gastroesophageal reflux disease. *Gastroenterol Clin North Am*. 1990;19:671–682.
3. Dent J, Brun J, Fendrick A, et al. An evidence-based appraisal of reflux disease management—the Genval Workshop Report. *Gut*. 1999;44:S1–S16.
4. Euler A, Byrne W. Twenty-four-hour esophageal intraluminal pH probe testing: a comparative analysis. *Gastroenterol*. 1981;80:957–961.
5. Richter J, Castell D. Gastroesophageal reflux. Pathogenesis, diagnosis, and therapy. *Ann Intern Med*. 1982;97:93–103.
6. Behar J, Biancani P, Sheahan D. Evaluation of esophageal tests in the diagnosis of reflux esophagitis. *Gastroenterol*. 1976;71:9–15.
7. Fass R, Fennerty M, Ofman J, et al. The clinical and economic value of a short course of omeprazole in patients with noncardiac chest pain. *Gastroenterol*. 1998;115:42–49.
8. Schenk B, Kuipers E, Klinkenberg-Knol E, et al. Omeprazole as a diagnostic tool in gastroesophageal reflux disease. *Am J Gastroenterol*. 1997;92:1997–2000.
9. Martinez S, Malagon I, Garewal H, Cui H, Fass R. Non-erosive reflux disease (NERD)—acid reflux and symptom patterns. *Aliment Pharmacol Ther*. 2003;17:537–545.
10. Schindlbeck N, Klauser A, Voderholzer W, Muller-Lissner S. Empiric therapy for gastroesophageal reflux disease. *Arch Intern Med*. 1995;155:1808–1812.
11. Johnsson F, Weywadt L, Solhaug J, Hernqvist H, Bengtsson L. One-week omeprazole treatment in the diagnosis of gastro-oesophageal reflux disease. *Scand J Gastroenterol*. 1998;33:15–20.
12. Fass R, Ofman J, Gralnek I, et al. Clinical and economic assessment of the omeprazole test in patients with symptoms suggestive of gastroesophageal reflux disease. *Arch Intern Med*. 1999;150:2161–2168.
13. Bate C, Riley S, Chapman R, Durnin A, Taylor M. Evaluation of omeprazole as a cost-effective diagnostic test for gastro-oesophageal reflux disease. *Aliment Pharmacol Ther*. 1999;13:59–66.
14. Juul-Hansen P, Rydning A, Jacobsen C, Hansen T. High-dose proton-pump inhibitors as a diagnostic test of gastroesophageal reflux disease in endoscopic-negative patients. *Scand J Gastroenterol*. 2001;36:806–810.
15. Squillace S, Young M, Sanowski R. Single dose omeprazole as a test for noncardiac chest pain (abstract). *Gastroenterol*. 1993;107:A197.
16. Young M, Sanowski R, Talbert G, Harrison M, Walker B. Omeprazole administration as a test for gastroesophageal reflux (abstract). *Gastroenterol*. 1992;102:192.
17. Pandak W, Arezo S, Everett S, et al. Short course of omeprazole: a better first diagnostic approach to noncardiac chest pain than endoscopy, manometry, or 24-hour esophageal pH monitoring. *J Clin Gastroenterol*. 2002;35:307–314.
18. Xia H, Lai K, Hu W, et al. Symptomatic response to lansoprazole predicts abnormal acid reflux in endoscopy-negative patients with non-cardiac chest pain. *Aliment Pharmacol Ther*. 2003;17:369–377.
19. Fass R, Pulliam G, Hayden C. Patients with non-cardiac chest pain (NCCP) receiving an empirical trial of high dose lansoprazole, demonstrate early symptom response—a double blind, placebo-controlled trial (abstract). *Gastroenterol*. 2001;120(A221):1162.
20. Fass R, Fullerton H, Hayden C, Garewal H. Patients with noncardiac chest pain (NCCP) receiving an empirical trial of high dose rabeprazole, demonstrate early symptom response—a double blind,

placebo-controlled trial (abstract). *Gastroenterol.* 2002;122(A580-A581):W1175.

21. Metz D, Childs M, Ruiz C, Weinstein G. Pilot study of the oral omeprazole test of reflux laryngitis. *Otolaryngol Head Neck Surg.* 1997;116:41-46.

22. Ours T, Kavuru M, Schilz R, Richter J. A prospective evaluation of esophageal testing and a double-blind, randomized study of omeprazole in a diagnostic and therapeutic algorithm for chronic cough. *Am J Gastroenterol.* 1999;94:3131-3138.

23. Jaspersen D, Diehl K, Geyer P, Martens E. Diagnostic omeprazole test in suspected reflux-associated chronic cough. *Pneumologie.* 1999;53:438-441.

24. Kiljander T, Salomaa E, Hietanen E, Terho E. Chronic cough and gastro-oesophageal reflux: a double-blind placebo-controlled study with omeprazole. *Eur Respir J.* 2000;16:633-638.

25. Fass R. Empirical trials in treatment of gastroesophageal reflux disease. *Dig Dis.* 2000;18:20-26.

26. Fass R, Ofman J, Sampliner R, Camargo L, Wendel C, Fennerty M. The omeprazole test is as sensitive as 24-h oesophageal pH monitoring in diagnosing gastro-oesophageal reflux disease in symptomatic patients with erosive oesophagitis. *Aliment Pharmacol Ther.* 2000;14:389-396.

27. Clouse R, Richter J, Heading R, Janssens J, Wilson J. Functional esophageal disorders. *Gut.* 1999;45(suppl 2):II31-36.

28. Fass R, Tougas G. Functional heartburn: the stimulus, the pain, and the brain. *Gut.* 2002;51:885-892.

29. Watson R, Tham T, Johnston B, McDougall N. Double blind cross-over placebo controlled study of omeprazole in the treatment of patients with reflux symptoms and physiological levels of acid reflux—the "sensitive oesophagus." *Gut.* 1997;40:587-590.

30. Numans M, Lau J, De Wit N, Bonis P. Short-term treatment with proton-pump inhibitors as a test for gastroesophageal reflux disease: a meta-analysis of diagnostic test characteristics. *Ann Intern Med.* 2004;140:518-527.

31. Lind T, Havelund T, Carlsson R, et al. Heartburn without oesophagitis: efficacy of omeprazole therapy and features determining therapeutic response. *Scand J Gastroenterol.* 1997;32(10):974-979.

32. Fass R, Malagon I, Schmulson M. Chest pain of esophageal origin. *Curr Opin Gastroenterol.* 2001;17:376-380.

33. Fass R. Noncardiac chest pain. In: Fass R, ed. *GERD/Dyspepsia: Fast facts.* Philadelphia, Pa: Hanley & Belfus; 2004: 183-196.

34. Locke G, III, Talley N, Fett S, Zinsmeister A, Melton L, III. Prevalence and clinical spectrum of gastroesophageal reflux: a population-based study in Olmsted County, Minnesota. *Gastroenterol.* 1997; 112:1448-1456.

35. Chambers J. Chest pain: heart, body or mind? *Psychosom Res.* 1997;43:161-165.

36. El-Serag H, Lee P, Buchner A, Inadomi J, Gavin M, McCarthy D. Lansoprazole treatment of patients with chronic idiopathic laryngitis: a placebo-controlled trial. *Am J Gastroenterol.* 2001;96:979-983.

37. Ofman J, Gralnek I, Udani J, Fennerty M, Fass R. The cost-effectiveness of the omeprazole test in patients with noncardiac chest pain. *Am J Med.* 1999;107: 219-227.

38. Ofman J, Dorn G, Fennerty M, Fass R. The clinical and economic impact of competing management strategies for gastro-oesophageal reflux disease. *Aliment Pharmacol Ther.* 2002;16:261-273.

39. Cremonini F, Wise J, Moayyedi P, Talley N. Meta-analysis: diagnostic and therapeutic use of proton pump inhibitors in non-cardiac chest pain. *Am J Gastroenterol.* 2005;100:1226-1232.

40. Dekel R, Martinez-Hawthorne S, Guillen R, Fass R. Evaluation of symptom index in identifying gastroesophageal reflux disease-related noncardiac chest pain. *J Clin Gastroenterol.* 2004;38:24-29.

41. Chambers J, R C, A A, Owen W. Effect of omeprazole in patients with chest pain and normal coronary anatomy: initial experience. *Int J Cardiol.* 1998;65:51–55.

42. Wang W, Huang J, Zheng G, et al. Is proton pump inhibitor testing an effective approach to diagnose gastroesophageal reflux disease in patients with noncardiac chest pain?: a meta-analysis. *Arch Intern Med.* 2005;165(11):1222–1228.

43. Fass R, Fennerty M, Johnson C, Camargo L, Sampliner R. Correlation of ambulatory 24-hour esophageal pH monitoring results in symptom improvement in patients with noncardiac chest pain due to gastroesophageal reflux disease. *J Clin Gastroenterol.* 1999;28:36–39.

44. Sontag S, O'Connell S, Khandelwal S, et al. Most asthmatics have gastroesophageal reflux with or without bronchodilator therapy. *Gastroenterol.* 1990;99:613–620.

45. Olson N. Laryngopharyngeal manifestations of gastroesophageal reflux disease. *Otolaryngol Clin North Am.* 1991;24:1201–1213.

46. Ott D, Ledbetter M, Koufman J, Chen M. Globus pharyngeus: radiographic evaluation and 24-hour pH monitoring of the pharynx and esophagus in 22 patients. *Radiology.* 1994;191:95–97.

47. McNally P, Maydonovitch C, Prosek R, Collette R, Wong R. Evaluation of gastroesophageal reflux as a case of idiopathic hoarseness. *Dig Dis Sci.* 1989;34:1900–1904.

48. Kamel P, Hanson D, Kahrilas P. Omeprazole for the treatment of posterior laryngitis. *Am J Med.* 1994;96:321–326.

49. Field S, Sutherland L. Does medical antireflux therapy improve asthma in asthmatics with gastroesophageal reflux?: a critical review of the literature. *Chest.* 1998;114:275–283.

50. Wo J, Grist W, Gussack G, Delgaudio J, Waring J. Empiric trial of high-dose omeprazole in patients with posterior laryngitis: a prospective study. *Am J Gastroenterol.* 1997;92:2160–2165.

51. Devault K, Castell D. Updated guidelines for the diagnosis and treatment of gastroesophageal reflux disease. The Practice Parameters Committee for the American College of Gastroenterology. *Am J Gastroenterol.* 1999;94:1434–1442.

52. Achem S, Kolts B, MacMath T, et al. Effects of omeprazole versus placebo in treatment of noncardiac chest pain and gastroesophageal reflux. *Dig Dis Sci.* 1997;42:2138–2145.

53. Harding S, Richter J, Guzzo M, Schan C, Alexander R, Bradle L. Asthma and gastroesophageal reflux: acid suppressive therapy improves asthma outcome. *Am J Med.* 1996;100:395–405.

CHAPTER 9

Brain Imaging in Noncardiac Chest Pain

Anthony R. Hobson
Qasim Aziz

Introduction

The esophagus is often considered a comparatively "simple" organ in the context of other gastrointestinal regions, which perform complex digestive functions. Whereas to some extent this is a valid opinion, abnormalities of esophageal function can lead to a wide array of debilitating symptoms such as dysphagia, heartburn, globus, odynophagia, and of course, pain. It is only when one attempts to explain the different mechanisms, which may lead to aberrant esophageal sensory signaling that the complexity of the esophageal sensory system is fully appreciated.

The aim of this chapter is to provide an overview of functional brain imaging data as it pertains to esophageal sensory processing: (1) in health, (2) during experimental paradigms aimed at modulating esophageal sensitivity, and (3) in patients with assumed esophageal pathology. We discuss how these studies have improved our understanding of esophageal-cortical signaling and how this has provided insights into mechanisms of esophageal hypersensitivity in NCCP.

Functional Brain Imaging Techniques

Four main functional brain imaging techniques have been used to assess esophageal sensory processing, positron emission tomography (PET), functional magnetic resonance imaging (fMRI), electroencephalography (EEG), and magnetoencephalography (MEG).

Each of these approaches has advantages and disadvantages, and importantly, are at their best when used to answer specific biological questions in homogeneous populations. It is not within the scope of this chapter to discuss the technical aspects of these different approaches. Where technical terms are used, the reader is referred to reviews of these different methodologies as we shall focus upon the physiologic relevance of these functional brain imaging studies.

Brain Regions Involved in Processing Esophageal Sensation

The first study to describe the cortical representation of esophageal sensation utilized PET and compared activation patterns to nonpainful and painful esophageal distension.[1] In this study the cortical regions involved in processing esophageal sensation were closely similar to those previously reported in studies of somatic pain.[1] In brief, nonpainful esophageal stimulation elicited bilateral activation of the primary (S1)/secondary (S2) somatosensory cortex and insula. As would be expected, painful esophageal stimulation increased activity within these regions but additionally activated the anterior cingulate cortex. This study gave us the first clue that visceral sensations were centrally processed in a manner closely similar to those from other body regions.

However, as esophageal pain has unique characteristics in comparison to pain arising for somatic structures such as the skin, several researchers explored whether the psychophysiological differences in the perception of these two sensory modalities could be explained by differences in cortical representation.

The cortical representation of esophageal sensation following nonpainful stim-

ulation of the proximal (somatic) and distal (visceral) esophagus was explored using fMRI.[2] Distension of the proximal esophagus was localized precisely to the upper chest and was represented in the trunk region of the left S1, whereas distension of the distal esophagus was perceived diffusely over the lower chest and represented bilaterally at the junction of S1 and S2. This was a fascinating if unsurprising observation which demonstrated that our ability to accurately localize bodily sensations requires discrete representation within the S1.

The novelty of this observation was that it provided objective evidence that the diffuse nature of visceral afferent innervation (discussed in more detail later) leads to diffuse activation of cortical regions that encode sensory discrimination. The implication of this was that visceral pain did not activate different brain regions when compared to somatic pain but merely that visceral pain activated the same region (S1) but did so over a more widely distributed spatial area. Different activation patterns were observed in the anterior cingulate gyrus with the proximal esophagus being represented in the right mid-anterior cingulate cortex (BA24) and the distal esophagus in the perigenual area (BA32). Differences in the activation of the dorsolateral prefrontal cortex and cerebellum were also observed for the two esophageal regions. These findings suggested that specialization in the sensory-discriminative, affective, and cognitive areas of the cortex accounted for the perceptual differences observed between the two sensory modalities.[2] An important caveat, however, was that the two stimuli were not balanced for factors such as unpleasantness and salience and therefore interpretation of these data remained guarded.

A more recent study performed by Strigo et al compared cortical activity generated by distension of the esophagus and thermal stimulation of the anterior chest wall.[3] In a well-designed study, both stimuli were matched psychophysically for intensity and area of stimulation (an 8-cm esophageal balloon and 9-cm thermal peltier device on the chest wall); however, esophageal stimulation was perceived to be more unpleasant than cutaneous stimulation. Interestingly, both esophageal and chest wall stimulation activated S1 in the region associated with the homuncular representation of the trunk; however, esophageal stimulation alone activated the more lateral aspects of S1 often referred to as gustatory region of S1 (Fig 9–1). The authors concluded that diffuse representation of the esophagus in S1 was consistent with the fact that visceral pain can be referred to the skin but not vice versa.

When taken in the context of the Aziz et al study,[1] these data also support the fact that pain fibers from somatic structures project to discrete regions within S1 whereas esophageal stimulation results in diffuse activation of afferents which project to multiple regions within S1. What these data also imply is that afferents from the esophagus converge with somatic afferents as they ascend to the brain and it is this convergence that explains the diffuse activity in S1.

Rather surprisingly, this study also revealed greater activation of the anterior portion of the insula (AI) to chest wall stimulation when compared to esophageal distension.[3] Previous studies have shown bilateral activation of the AI to be the most consistent finding across all esophageal neuroimaging studies[4] and this area plays an important role in the emotional modulation of esophageal

sensory processing.[5] However, AI is also strongly activated by thermal stimulation[6] and the differences seen here may in part reflect the fact that a higher number of somatic thermosensitive neurons are present in this region when compared to visceral specific neurons. Both stimuli produced bilateral activation of the posterior insula, which is known to process somesthetic and painful sensations,[7] providing further evidence for the convergence of visceral and somatic pain processing.

In summary, esophageal sensation and pain is processed within a network of cortical and subcortical structures similar to those activated by stimulation of other bodily structures such as the skin. No cortical region has been identified which is specific to visceral/esophageal sensory processing and all the data reported at present points to the fact that esophageal pain is just one part of the pain continuum with differences observed related to the unique innervation of this region. The following section provides further evidence for this observation.

Characterizing Extrinsic Esophageal Afferent Pathways and Cortical Neural Activity in Real Time

Images obtained with metabolic imaging techniques such as PET and fMRI provide excellent neuroanatomic information and, with careful design, experiments can begin to tease out different aspects of sensory and pain processing. The major limitation of these two techniques is their temporal resolution, that is, how quickly the measured signal occurs following the

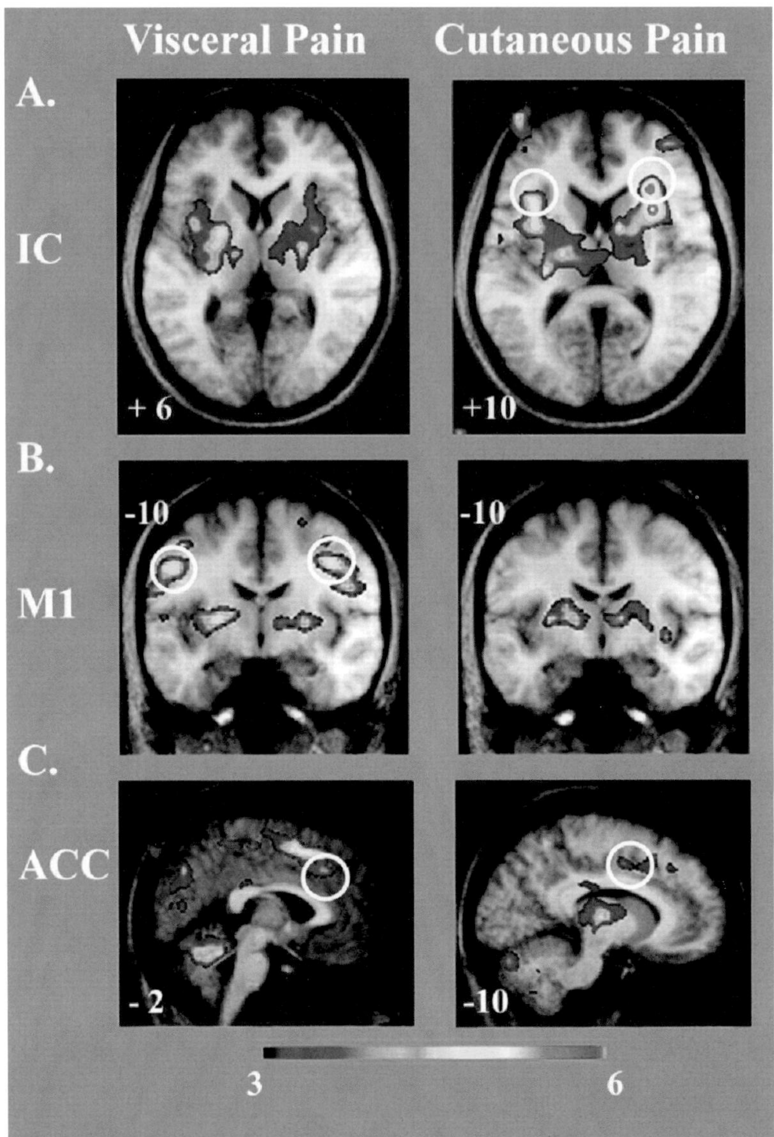

Fig 9–1. Cortical activation evoked by noxious esophageal distension and noxious thermal heat in insular cortex (*A;* IC), primary motor cortex (*B;* M1), and anterior cingulate cortex (*C;* ACC). A. Noxious cutaneous but not visceral stimulation resulted in significantly higher activity in the right anterior insula ($p < 0.05$, paired *t*-test) with a similar tendency in the left anterior insula ($p = 0.1$, paired *t*-test). **B.** Noxious visceral but not cutaneous stimulation significantly activated primary motor cortex (M1, face area) on the right ($p < 0.05$) with a similar tendency on the left ($p = 0.1$, paired *t*-test). **C.** Noxious visceral and cutaneous stimulation showed differential activation within ACC with visceral distention represented more anteriorly. (Reproduced with permission from Strigo et al, Figure 3 in *J Neurophysiol.* 2003 Jun;89(6):3294–3303.)

stimulus and how sensitive this signal is to rapid changes in the environmental setting or to the stimulus characteristics. This is not a problem if the parameters you are measuring are tonic such as an acidic infusion, for instance, or occur over several seconds such as responding to visual cues (see next section for more details).

However, one of the fundamental questions required to understand the etiology of symptoms in conditions such as NCCP is whether the problem is related to increased sensitivity of esophageal afferents or whether this condition is predominantly driven by psychological factors. To discriminate between these two possible physiologic drivers requires the ability to record neural responses as they occur in real time. Metabolic imaging techniques cannot provide this degree of resolution and therefore researchers have turned to techniques such as magneto- (MEG) and electroencephalography (EEG).

EEG measures the brain's electrical activity via electrodes placed on the scalp, whereas MEG records the minute magnetic fields generated by activated groups of cortical neurons via exquisitely sensitive sensors submersed in a liquid helium-filled helmet placed on the subject's head. Both techniques have millisecond temporal resolution; however, MEG is able to accurately localize cortical activity to within 5 mm as the magnetic field MEG measures passes through the skull without distortion. EEG has a poorer spatial resolution (1–2 cm) as the electrical field generated within the brain meets resistance on its passage to the surface in the form of structures such as the skull, meninges, and scalp which lie between the cortical source and the recording electrode. EEG is much more readily available and as with all of these approaches, one must balance between

what is desirable, what is achievable, and what is necessary to address specific biological questions.

The most common methodology used to assess esophageal afferent function with MEG and EEG has been the evoked response paradigm.[8-16] Here a repeated stimulus is applied to the esophagus which is abrupt in its onset (electrical stimulation or rapid mechanical distension using custom-built inflation devices) and short in its duration (>1 second). The rapid stimulus triggers an ascending afferent volley which is transmitted proximally via vagal and spinal pathways to higher cortical structures. Within these structures, electromagnetic fluctuations occur in response to the arrival of the stimulus and subsequent processing of this information.

The recorded signal is small when compared to the brain's ongoing electrical activity but because it occurs at the same moment in time following each stimulus averaging these responses reduces the randomly occurring brain activity and enhances the stimulus-specific related activity. The final recorded waveform comprises a sequence of negative and positive reflections, with each peak/ trough corresponding to a specific step in the processing sensory information. An example, of such a waveform is given in Figure 9–2.

Using EEG, it is possible to gain some information about the underlying cortical sources that generate the recorded waveform by using multiple sensors on the scalp. In 1995, Aziz et al[8] reported data on cortical potentials evoked (CEP) by balloon distension of the proximal and distal esophagus in healthy volunteers. Esophageal evoked cortical potentials were recorded in all subjects with an initial negative and positive component

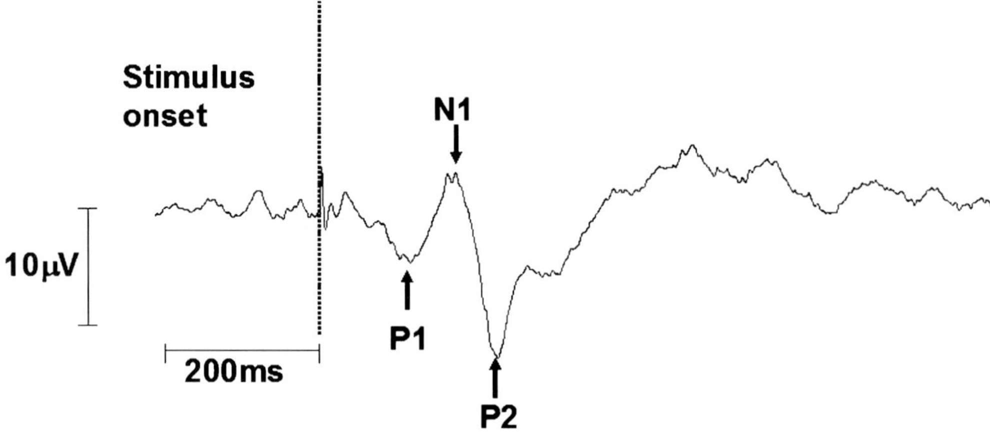

Fig 9–2. A typical esophageal CEP response recorded in a healthy subject in response to 200 electrical stimuli. The three components labeled P1, N1 and P2 reflect the stimulus-specific cortical activity which occurs in the first 300 ms following a stimulus. Later activity is also sometimes observed and this reflects endogenous brain activity.

(N1 and P1), followed by a second negative and positive component (N2 and P2). The morphology and the scalp topography of the N1 component elicited by proximal and distal esophageal stimulation suggested activation of the primary somatosensory cortex and/or the insular. There was also evidence for hemispheric dominance for the N1 potential which was independent of handedness. The frontal emphasis of the proximal esophageal N1 component, in contrast to the central emphasis of the distal esophageal N1 component, suggested that different neuronal populations were activated by stimulation of the two sites.[8] This was subsequently proven to be the case in the study using fMRI as discussed in the previous section, a good example of how different brain imaging approaches can provide complementary information.[2] With metabolic imaging techniques becoming more accessible, researchers using the CEP response concentrated less on spatial localization and more on characterizing the properties of esophageal affer-

ent pathways, and this is really where the technique came into its own.

Frieling et al were the first to record EP responses to esophageal stimulation and they, along with other investigators, suggested that the esophageal CEP was predominantly mediated via vagal afferent pathways.[9] However, further studies revealed that as stimulation intensity and sensory perception increased toward pain, there was an associated reduction in the latency and increase in amplitude of the CEP components.[15] This phenomenon is common across all evoked potential modalities and reflects the recruitment of an increasing number of afferents. The stimulus response characteristics of the CEP therefore implicate spinal afferents in the mediation of this response as most studies show that vagal afferents saturate at stimulation levels well below the noxious range.[17]

Importantly, the ability to record objective neurophysiologic measures which correspond directly to subjective pain ratings overcomes many of the limitations of previous studies of visceral hypersensitivity which rely on descriptive methods of sensory reporting. Elimination of subjective factors that introduce response bias is difficult and no truly objective measures of visceral sensation have been available until CEP, the importance of which will become more apparent in the clinical section of this chapter.

A comparison of esophageal CEP elicited by electrical and mechanical stimulation showed that both responses were mediated by thinly myelinated Aδ-fibers, both produced responses of identical morphology, and that the latency difference between the first mechanical and electrical EEP component of approximately 50 ms was due to the physical delay encountered during balloon inflation not activation of different fiber types. This is not to say that unmyelinated C-fibers are not activated by esophageal stimulation, just that they do not contribute to the early response complex recorded with this type of CEP paradigm.[14]

Importantly, the amplitude of mechanically evoked esophageal CEP was smaller than that seen by electrical stimulation. It is known that the amplitude of the esophageal CEP increases with increased afferent recruitment. These amplitude differences could therefore be explained by the fact that mechanical stimulation is specific to mechanosensitive afferent receptors whereas electrical stimulation activated all afferents regardless of modality, hence leading to greater afferent recruitment.[14]

Interestingly, visceral CEP, in general, are similar in nature to somatic pain CEP responses elicited by thermal cutaneous laser stimulation. Like esophageal stimulation, laser stimulation selectively activates nociceptive afferents, namely, thinly myelinated Aδ and unmyelinated C-fibers.

The resultant laser CEP response shares several other characteristics with visceral CEP in that it habituates over time, is maximally recorded at the vertex, and changes in the latency of components can occur with alteration of the level of vigilance/attention afforded to the stimulus.[18] These similarities become important when considering the physiologic basis and functional relevance of the CEP and also provide additional evidence to that presented earlier which supports the fact that visceral pain is *not* unique but one part of the pain continuum.

A further piece of evidence to support this concept comes from our own MEG studies. We recently performed a series of experiments to characterize the temporal sequence of brain activation following painful stimulation of the esophagus and extrapolated these data to the CEP response. It has been shown that in a manner similar to somatic pain, esophageal pain is initially processed in parallel within the S1, S2, and the posterior insular (PI) cortex.[13] Once again it has been demonstrated that unlike painful activation of a limb, which predominantly activates contralateral S1, esophageal electrical stimulation activates S1 bilaterally in both trunk and intra-abdominal homuncular regions. Later activation occurs in brain regions which process affective aspects of pain such as the cingulate and anterior insula cortices. Extrapolation of these data to the scalp-recorded CEP response allowed us to demonstrate that the initial P1 component which occurs approximately 80 msec following the stimulus, reflects activation of these primary and secondary somatosensory areas. The middle latency N1 and P2 components appear to reflect an amalgamation of cortical activity within sensory and affective brain regions.[13]

We were also able to dissociate brain activity specific to the stimulus from that which was endogenously produced in relation to the stimulus. This is probably the most important feature of CEP as it allows us to differentiate between brain activities that provide information about the level of sensitivity within the ascending (peripheral) afferent pathway from that generated endogenously in response to the stimulus. In a previous study by Hollerbach et al, it was clearly shown that in the absence of a peripheral stimulus the early P1/N1/P2 complex cannot be elicited.[19] However, if the subject is anticipating a stimulus and this stimulus is skipped, then the subject still engages higher order brain processes and the late response (>300 msec) is apparent in the tracings[19] and our data supported this finding.

The conclusion that can be drawn from this section is that CEP/MEG are currently the only techniques available that allow for objective measures of esophageal afferent pathway sensitivity. This is obviously an important point to grasp as the treatment strategies of patients could be tailored to attenuate the appropriate aberrant mechanism if such clinical evidence were routinely obtained. The next section provides an insight into the effects of experimental sensitization of esophageal afferent pathways.

How Does Experimental Esophageal Acidification Affect Esophageal Afferent Pathways and Cortical Processing?

The esophagus is continually bathed in irritants either ingested or refluxed by the host. One mechanism that may lead to inappropriate signaling of these esophageal sensory events is increased esophageal afferent sensitivity. Experimentally, it has been consistently shown that short duration esophageal acidification can lead to persistent increases in esophageal sensitivity to a range of sensory modalities.[20,21]

For example, it has recently been demonstrated that in health, short duration esophageal acidification (5 minutes) can lead to transient reductions in esophageal pain thresholds to electrical stimulation. A second 5-minute acid infusion given 1 hour following the first induces a much greater and more prolonged reduction in esophageal pain thresholds and this response is exaggerated in patients with NCCP.[21] A series of studies by several groups have indicated that central sensitization of esophageal spinal dorsal horn neurons appears to be a likely mechanism in the development and maintenance of acid-induced hypersensitivity in this type of model, and it is plausible that such a mechanism contributes to symptoms in NCCP and other esophageal disorders such as functional heartburn.

Objective mechanistic evidence to support the role of increased esophageal afferent pathway sensitivity in a model of esophageal acidification comes from a study which recorded esophageal CEPs prior to and following a 30-minute acid infusion. This study showed that despite using the same sensory stimulus to evoke pre- and postinfusion CEP responses, following acid and not saline, CEP responses were potentiated.[22]

This study has been replicated by a second group[23] and similar studies using fMRI have recently provided complementary evidence to support the notion that experimental esophageal acidification can amplify central signaling of both innocuous and liminal inputs.[20] Kern et al studied 11 gastroesophageal reflux disease (GERD) patients and 15 healthy controls with fMRI. Activity was recorded twice in each subject, during two 5-minute intervals of 0.1N HCl, separated by 5 minutes of NaCl perfusion.

The major findings of this study were that the time between when GERD patients reported feeling heartburn in response to the acid infusion to the instant of fMRI signal increase averaged 1.60 ± 0.80 and 1.85 ± 0.60 min, respectively. Average maximum percent signal increase in the GERD patients ($16.3 \pm 3.5\%$) was significantly greater than that of healthy controls ($3.8 \pm 0.9\%; p < 0.01$). Interestingly, the temporal fMRI signal characteristics during heartburn were significantly different from those of subliminal acid stimulation in controls.

This study showed that whereas cortical activity associated with perceived and unperceived esophageal acid exposure involves similar brain regions, it occurs more rapidly and with greater intensity in GERD patients than the activity in response to subliminal acid exposure in healthy controls.[20] This finding further supports the role increased central afferent signaling plays in GERD and in esophageal hypersensitivity.

The mounting evidence to support the role of central sensitization-mediated increased esophageal afferent pathway sensitivity as an important mechanism of esophageal hypersensitivity comes from CEP studies in patients with nonerosive reflux disease (NERD). In the first pilot study in our laboratory, it was shown that esophageal sensitivity to electrical stimulation was significantly correlated with acid reflux as determined by ambulatory pH recordings.[24] These data showed

that as the DeMeester score increased this was associated with an increase in esophageal pain thresholds. This group of 15 NERD patient were then separated into reflux-negative and reflux-positive subgroups and it was shown that despite using significantly lower stimulation intensities to elicit esophageal CEP in reflux-negative patients equivalent amplitude and latency responses were recorded when compared to reflux-positive patients.[24]

These data were further supported by a study of Yang et al which described enhanced esophageal CEP to mechanical esophageal stimulation in 21 patients with functional heartburn when compared to healthy subjects. Equivalent or enhanced CEP responses to reduced esophageal afferent input strongly supports the hypothesis that increased afferent pathway sensitivity contributes to esophageal hypersensitivity in NERD, at least in a subset of patients.[25]

How Does Psychological Modulation Change the Way that Esophageal Afferent Information Is Processed by the Brain?

The affective dimension of pain combines the degree of unpleasantness perceived with the emotions associated with its appraisal and future implications. It has long been recognized that cognitive modulation of pain can have dramatic effects on its perception. There is a high incidence (50–80%) of psychological disorders such as heightened anxiety, depression, somatization, dysthymia, and panic disorders reported in conditions such as NCCP (see chapter 6 for more details). Therefore, a natural progression for researchers working in the esophageal pain area was to examine the effects that different psychological states have on the distribution and intensity of cortical activation using brain imaging.

One such study examined the role of negative emotional context on the processing of esophageal sensation. Psychologists have long noted that facial expressions can provide the emotional context to our environment in which we receive information. For instance, information received while observing a facial expression of fear would associate it with a negative emotional context, whereas a smiling face would produce association with a positive emotional context. Therefore, this study examined the effects of negative and neutral emotional states on the processing and perception of nonpainful esophageal distension.[5]

The study revealed that esophageal distension presented during a negative emotional context was perceived more intensely, induced greater anxiety, and was associated with increased cortical activity within the anterior insula and dorsal anterior cingulate cortex, when compared to distension presented during neutral emotional context.

These findings provided additional evidence to support the fact that changes in the pattern of cortical activity could be directly associated with psychophysiologic changes, which was important as it helped to validate the use of brain imaging in identifying mechanisms of esophageal sensory dysfunction. Importantly, as many NCCP patients are anxious, depressed, and associate esophageal/chest sensations with negative feelings, these findings provide evidence that psychological factors *could* increase our sensitivity to innocuous sensations.

In another study, the role that attentional state plays in modifying pain was

examined.[26] Experiments have shown that pain is perceived as less intense when we are distracted from it and more intense when we focus our attention upon it. In conditions such as irritable bowel syndrome, it has been shown that patients often selectively attend to sensations that arise from the gut and that this is an important factor in sustaining symptoms.[27]

As esophageal sensations rarely breach our consciousness in health, it may be expected that when they do arise, processing of this sensory information may demand increased attentional resources when compared to sensory input from other modalities. This was demonstrated in a study that compared cortical activation patterns in response to nonpainful esophageal stimulus with those that occurred following a visual stimulus. Selectively focusing attention on esophageal stimuli activated regions of the brain involved in processing sensory information (S1 and S2) as well as cognitive and emotional regions (ACC and insula). In contrast, activation related to visual stimuli was restricted to the visual cortex.[27]

Interestingly, when selectively attending to a visual stimulus, the cortical response to esophageal distension was significantly attenuated.[27] This implies that if we focus attention on GI sensations, as often occurs in functional pain syndromes, additional neural resources are allocated to processing of this information. This may lead to an amplification of innocuous sensory events resulting in increased awareness and exaggerated emotional responsiveness. It is conceivable that such a process occurs in some NCCP patients and may partly explain the heightened sensory responsiveness observed in response to experimental stimuli in many clinical studies.

The role of anticipation in pain experiments has been examined in several studies and these have demonstrated that some of the cortical regions implicated specifically in pain processing may, in fact, be neural correlates related to the anticipation of an imminently painful event.[28] A recent study which used a pavlovian, classical conditioning paradigm to examine the effects of such factors on esophageal sensory processing revealed that the majority of cortical regions activated by esophageal stimulation are also activated by the anticipation of such a stimulus.

In this experiment, subjects learned to associate a visual cue with a painful esophageal stimulus. After this initial learning phase, subjects were presented with the visual cue but the esophageal stimulation did not occur. Despite the lack of stimulation, activation was seen in S1, S2, ACC, insula, and prefrontal cortex. As the subject began to realize that the visual cue was no longer linked to esophageal pain (extinction phase), there was a linear decrease in activity within these regions.[29] This once again showed that the anticipatory/cognitive components of brain activity observed during pain experiments have to be taken into account when using brain imaging and supports the use of EEG/MEG which have the temporal resolution to achieve this.

Can We Construct a Hypothetical Model of Esophageal Sensory Processing that is Relevant to NCCP?

Considering all of the information presented above we can begin to understand what happens when a sensory impulse is transmitted from the esophagus and processed within the brain. The esophageal afferent nerves are few in number when compared to other types of afferents within the spinal cord, but diverge as they leave the esophagus entering the spinal cord at multiple levels. Here they converge with somatic afferents as a way of amplifying the signal and ascend to the thalamus and onto higher cortical regions. The fact that the esophageal afferent information has "piggybacked" onto somatic afferent is reflected by the diffuse activation of S1 in particular, which most results in the diffuse perception of esophageal sensation.

Further amplification of the sensory signal may occur if central sensitization develops, enlarging the receptive fields of spinal afferents and increasing the number of afferents recruited by the esophageal input. Alternatively, amplification may occur at higher cortical levels as more neural resources are allocated to signals arriving from this particular body region. Here the sensory signal arriving in the cortex is normal but the brain's enhanced endogenous response to its arrival leads to increased perception. The big question, therefore, is do these two proposed mechanisms contribute to esophageal hypersensitivity in NCCP?

We have recently provided preliminary evidence to support the hypothesis that subsets exist within the NCCP population which have esophageal hypersensitivity and neurophysiologic profiles that have characteristics of both aberrant mechanisms. In this study, we showed that in one subset of NCCP patients, esophageal hypersensitivity as determined by reduced esophageal pain threshold to electrical stimulation was associated with enhanced (or equivalent) early CEP components when compared to controls. This indicated that despite using reduced sensory input to trigger the afferent response, the resultant signal arriving in the brain was increased when compared to normal, indicating that increased afferent pathway sensitivity.[30]

In a second subset of NCCP patients with esophageal hypersensitivity, the early CEP components were attenuated when compared to controls. This indicated that the afferent signal arriving in the cortex was normal, thus providing no evidence of increased afferent pathway sensitivity in this subset of patients. Although the early CEP components appeared attenuated, they were probably normal given the fact that the intensity of stimulation was lower than would be used in a control subject. However, the late endogenous component of the CEP was enhanced in many of these patients, and this provided evidence that the amplification of esophageal sensory information occurred after its arrival in the brain, supporting the role of psychological factors in esophageal hypersensitivity.[30] Illustrations of these two distinct phenotypic representations can be seen in Figure 9-3.

Summary and Future Direction

To summarize, with regard to understanding esophageal sensory signaling and mechanisms of esophageal hypersensitivity, we have come a long way in the last decade. Furthermore we have evidence of different phenotypic characteristics within the NCCP population. We also have a battery of quantitative sensory testing techniques to probe esophageal afferents, psychological assessments to probe individual traits, and a combination of functional brain imaging methodologies that provide detailed and objective measures of afferent activity and cortical

processing. The question remains, how will this progress translate into effective treatments for NCCP patients?

What Should We Do Next?

Positive drug effects in studies of visceral hypersensitivity are often diluted by patient heterogeneity. A compound with antihyperalgesic properties will only be effective in patients with afferent sensitization. As stated earlier in this chapter, conventional sensory testing cannot differentiate between hyperalgesia caused by afferent sensitization from that caused by psychological factors (stress, for example).

CEP have been used in studies of central *somatic* pain to dissociate these two mechanisms[31] and our recent study has shown that CEP can be used in a similar fashion in patients with esophageal pain.[30] This study showed that only 30% of patients recruited using standard inclusion diagnostic criteria for NCCP had afferent sensitization. Hypothetically, this would mean that an antihyperalgesic compound would not be of benefit beyond placebo in nearly 70% of patients recruited into a clinical trial. Therefore, incorporating an objective measure of central afferent processing into existing pain models would greatly improve the sensitivity of the study and interpretation of the clinical outcome measures. Conversely, those patients with evidence of altered endogenous cortical processing of esophageal sensory information or psychological disorders would benefit from treatments which target this mechanism. We propose, that over the next few years, small clinical trials should utilize the tools at our disposal and treat the pathophysiology present in individual

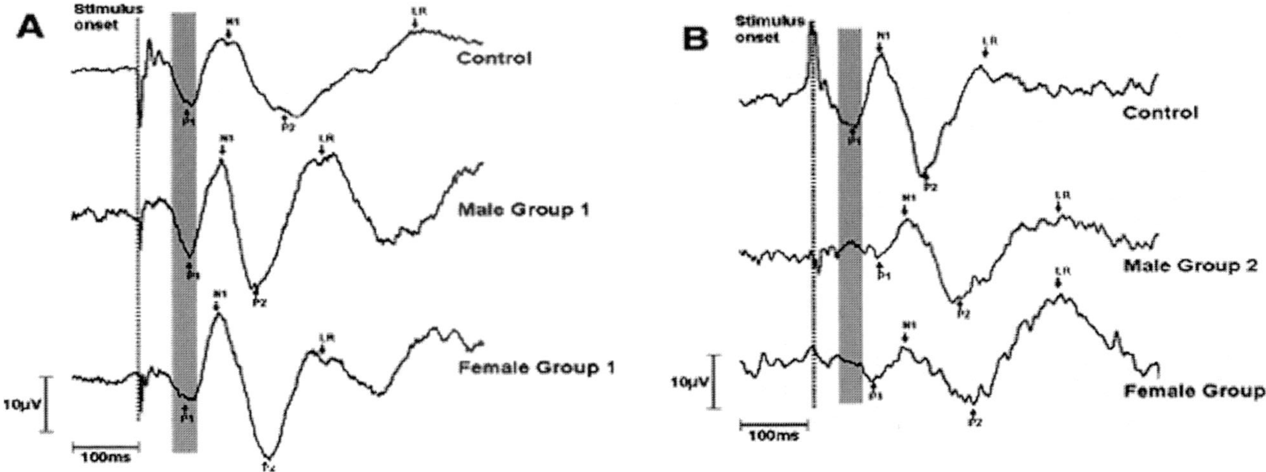

Fig 9–3. Panel A shows esophageal CEP responses in a control participant (*top trace*) and 2 NCCP patients with increased afferent pathway sensitivity (*group 1: middle and bottom traces*). Despite group 1 patients having significantly lower esophageal pain thresholds (PTs) when compared with control (75 vs 45 and 35 mA), the CEP response is equivalent in terms of both amplitude and latency (as indicated by the gray shaded region for P1). This indicates increased afferent pathway sensitivity in this subgroup of NCCP patients. In panel B CEP responses in a control participant (*top trace*) and 2 NCCP patients with attenuated early CEP components (*group 2: middle and bottom traces*) are shown. Although group 2 patients also have significantly lower esophageal PTs when compared with control (63 vs 42 and 37 mA, respectively), the latency of the CEP components are delayed (as indicated by the gray shaded region for P1). This indicates that increased pain sensitivity in this subgroup of NCCP patients is not associated with increased afferent pathway sensitivity. (Reproduced with permission from Hobson et al, *Gastroenterology.* 2006 Jan;130(1):80–88.)

patients rather than their unsatisfactory diagnosis. Translating our knowledge into successful treatment strategies in NCCP should be our next goal and one which should be undertaken with common sense and vigor.

References

1. Aziz Q, Andersson JL, Valind S, et al. Identification of human brain loci processing esophageal sensation using positron emission tomography. *Gastroenterology.* 1997; 113(1):50-59.

2. Aziz Q, Thompson DG, Ng VW, et al. Cortical processing of human somatic and visceral sensation. *J Neurosci.* 2000; 20(7):2567-2663.

3. Strigo IA, Duncan GH, Boivin M, Bushnell MC. Differentiation of visceral and cutaneous pain in the human brain. *J Neurophysiol.* 2003;89(6):3294-3303.

4. Derbyshire SW. A systematic review of neuroimaging data during visceral stimulation. *Am J Gastroentrol.* 2003;98(1): 12-20.

5. Phillips ML, Gregory LJ, Cullen S, et al. The effect of negative emotional context on neural and behavioural responses to oesophageal stimulation. *Brain.* 2003; 126(pt 3):669-684l; erratum in *Brain.* 2003;126(pt 5):1248.

6. Casey KL, Minoshima S, Morrow TJ, Koeppe RA. Comparison of human cerebral activation pattern during cutaneous warmth, heat pain, and deep cold pain. *J Neurophysiol.* 1996;76(1):571-581.

7. Frot M, Mauguiere F. Operculo-insular responses to nociceptive skin stimulation in humans. A review of the literature. [in French]. *Neurophysiol Clin.* 1999;29(5): 401-410.

8. Aziz Q, Furlong PL, Barlow J, et al. Topographic mapping of cortical potentials evoked by distension of the human prox-

imal and distal oesophagus. *Electroencephalogr Clin Neurophysiol.* 1995;96(3): 219-228,

9. Frieling T, Enck P, Wienbeck M. Cerebral responses evoked by electrical stimulation of the esophagus in normal subjects. *Gastroenterology.* 1989;97(2):475-478.

10. Frobert O, Arendt-Neilsen L, Bak P, Funch-Jensen P, Bagger J. Electrical stimulation of the esophageal mucosa: Perception and brain evoked potentials. *Scand J Gastroenterol.* 1994;29(9):776-781.

11. Furlong PL, Aziz Q, Singh KD, Thompson DG, Hobson A, Harding GF. Cortical localisation of magnetic fields evoked by oesophageal distension. *Electroencephalogr.* 1998;108(3):234-243.

12. Hecht M, Kober H, Claus D, Hilz M, Vieth J, Neundorfer B. The electrical and magnetical cerebral responses evoked by electrical stimulation of the esophagus and the location of their cerebral sources. *Clin Neurophysiol.* 1999;110(8):1435-1444.

13. Hobson AR, Furlong PL, Worthen SF, et al. Real-time imaging of human cortical activity evoked by painful esophageal stimulation. *Gastroenterology.* 2005;128(3): 610-619.

14. Hobson AR, Sarkar S, Furlong PL, Thompson DG, Aziz Q. A cortical evoked potential study of afferents mediating human esophageal sensation. *Am J Physiol Gastrointest Liver Physiol.* 2000;279(1): G139-G147.

15. Hollerbach S, Kamath MV, Chen Y, Fitzpatrick D, Upton AR, Tougas G. The magnitude of the central response to esophageal electrical stimulation is intensity dependent. *Gastroenterology.* 1997; 112(4):1137-1146.

16. Loose R, Schnitzler A, Sarkar S, et al. Cortical activation during mechanical oesophagus stimulation: A neuromagnetic study. *Neurogastroenterol Motil.* 1999;11(3): 163-171.

17. Sengupta JN, Kauvar D, Goyal RK. Characteristics of vagal esophageal tension-sensitive afferent fibers in the opossum. *J Neurophysiol.* 1989;61(5):1001-1010.

18. Arendt Nielsen L. Characteristics, detection, and modulation of laser-evoked vertex potentials. *Acta Anesthesiol Scand Suppl.* 1994;101:7–44.

19. Hollerbach S, Fitzpatrick D, Shine G, Kamath MV, Upton AR, Tougas G. Cognitive evoked potentials to anticipated oesophageal stimulus in humans: quantitative assessment of the cognitive aspects of visceral perception. *Neurogastroenterol Motil.* 1999;11(1):37–46.

20. Kern MK, Birn RM, Jaradeh S, et al. Identification and characterization of cerebral cortical response to esophageal mucosal acid exposure and distention. *Gastroenterology.* 1998;115(6):1353–1362.

21. Sarkar S, Aziz Q, Woolf CJ, Hobson AR, Thompson DG. Contribution of central sensitisation to the development of non-cardiac chest pain. *Lancet.* 2000; 356(9236):115–119.

22. Sarkar S, Hobson AR, Furlong PL, Woolf CJ, Thompson DG, Aziz Q. Central neural mechanisms mediating human visceral hypersensitivity. *Am J Physiol Gastrointest Liver Physiol.* 2001;281(5):G1196–G1202.

23. Sami SA, Rossel P, Dimcevski G, et al. Cortical changes to experimental sensitization of the human esophagus. *Neuroscience.* 2006;140:269–279.

24. Hobson AR, Furlong P, Aziz Q. The role of esophageal afferent pathway sensitivity in non-erosive reflux disease [abstract]. *Gastroenterology.* 2004;

25. Yang M, Li ZS, Xu XR, et al. Characterization of cortical potentials evoked by oesophageal balloon distention and acid perfusion in patients with functional heartburn. *Neurogastroenterol Motil.* 2006;18:292–299.

26. Gregory LJ, Yaguez L, Williams SC, et al. Cognitive modulation of the cerebral processing of human oesophageal sensation using functional magnetic resonance imaging. *Gut.* 2003;52(12):1671–1677.

27. Whitehead WE, Palsson OS. Is rectal pain sensitivity a biological marker for irritable bowel syndrome: psychological influences on pain perception. *Gastroenterology.* 1998;115(5):1263–1271.

28. Ploghaus A, Tracey I, Gati J, et al. Dissociating pain from its anticipation in the human brain. *Science.* 1999;284(5422): 1979–1981.

29. Yaguez L, Coen S, Gregory LJ, et al. Brain response to visceral aversive conditioning: a functional magnetic resonance imaging study. *Gastroenterology.* 2005; 128(7):1819–1820.

30. Hobson AR, Furlong PL, Sarkar S, et al. Neurophysiologic assessment of esophageal sensory processing in noncardiac chest pain. *Gastroenterology.* 2006; 130(1):80–88.

31. Garcia-Larrea L, Peyron R, Laurent B, Mauguiere F. Association and dissociation between laser-evoked potentials and pain perception. *Neuroreport.* 1997;8(17): 3875–3789.

CHAPTER 10

Noncardiac Chest Pain– Treatment

Michael Shapiro
Anmarie Easley Moore
Ronnie Fass

Introduction

Treatment for noncardiac chest pain (NCCP) should be tailored to patients' potential underlying mechanisms. However, the different causes of NCCP are not fully understood and often overlap clinically. Important etiologic factors include: gastroesophageal reflux disease (GERD), esophageal dysmotility, visceral hyperalgesia, autonomic dysfunction, and psychological comorbidity.

GERD is by far the most common cause and may be present in up to 60% of the patients with NCCP.[1] Although the presence of abnormal esophageal acid exposure on 24-hour pH testing and/or esophageal mucosal injury on upper endoscopy are suggestive of GERD, only symptom improvement during acid suppressive therapy strongly supports a causal relationship. To date, proton-pump inhibitors (PPIs) are the mainstay therapy for GERD-related NCCP. Additionally, high-dose PPI therapy given over a short period of time may serve as a highly sensitive, specific, and cost-effective method for diagnosing GERD-related NCCP.[2] Patients responsive to the PPI test should be treated with a PPI, at least double dose, for an additional period of 2 to 3 months (Fig 10–1). Subsequently, patients may attempt to taper down the PPI dose to once a day. However, in most patients with GERD-related NCCP, long-term treatment with a PPI is usually required for the prevention of symptoms relapse.

In those patients who are not responsive to high-dose PPI, esophageal manometry should be considered. Currently, the role of esophageal manometry in patients with NCCP is limited to the diagnosis of achalasia, which has a specific therapy.

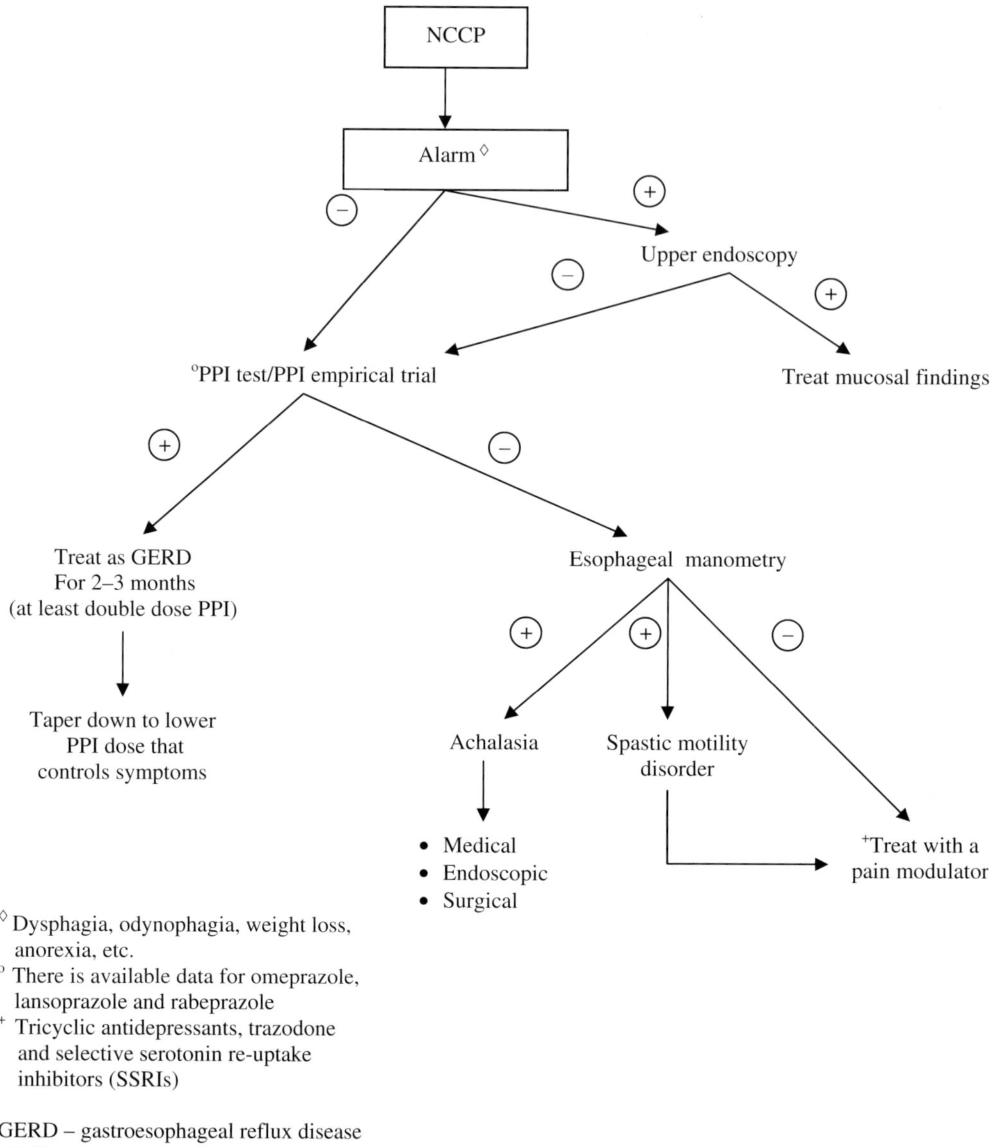

Fig 10–1. Diagnostic and treatment algorithm for NCCP.

In patients with other spastic motility disorders, pain modulators appear to provide better symptom control when compared to muscle relaxants. Additionally, in patients with functional chest pain of presumed esophageal origin (without esophageal dysmotility), pain modulators are the cornerstone of therapy.

The pain modulators that have been assessed in NCCP patients include tricyclic antidepressants (TCAs), trazodone, selective serotonin reuptake inhibitors

(SSRIs), octreotide, and theophylline. TCAs are the most commonly used pain modulators in clinical practice. Because of the varied effect of TCAs on the different target receptors, failure of oneTCA to improve symptoms is not indicative of future failure of other TCAs.

Novel therapies with visceral analgesic properties are emerging and may be clinically available in the near future. The most promising are the partial $5HT_4$ agonists, $5HT_3$ antagonists, kappa agonists, and others.

The high prevalence of psychological comorbidity in patients with NCCP is the impetus for adding psychiatric evaluation and intervention to the current therapeutic armamentarium of NCCP. Although a variety of pharmacologic and nonpharmacologic modalities have been assessed, psychological evaluation and possible intervention should always be considered in patients who appear to be refractory to medical treatment.

GERD-Related NCCP

Treatment for GERD-related NCCP includes lifestyle modifications (Table 10–1) and pharmacologic intervention (Table 10–2). Antireflux surgery and endoscopic therapy are not commonly used.

Lifestyle Modifications

Elevation of the head of the bed, weight loss, smoking cessation, avoidance of alcohol, coffee, citrus, and other food products that can exacerbate symptoms of gastroesophageal reflux as well as other lifestyle modifications are widely used

Table 10–1. Lifestyle Modifications for GERD

- Avoid medications that exacerbate gastroesophageal reflux: anticholinergics, tricyclics and other antidepressants, calcium channel blockers, and benzodiazepines.
- Avoid smoking or drinking alcohol.
- Avoid eating large fatty meals, spicy food, chocolate, peppermint, coffee, onions, and citrus juices.
- Avoid carbonated beverages.
- Reduce weight (if overweight).
- Avoid tight-fitting garments.
- Elevate the head of the bed.
- Avoid assuming the supine position up to 3 hours after a meal.

and considered by many physicians as an integral component of any therapeutic intervention in GERD.[3,4] However, data supporting the usefulness of lifestyle modifications in GERD are relatively scant and specifically in GERD-related NCCP are still unavailable. Regardless, enthusiasm about lifestyle modifications in general is so prevalent among physicians that many of the GERD-related NCCP patients are likely to receive a full or partial list to follow in addition to other therapeutic modalities (see Table 10–1). There is very little information about the long-term compliance of patients with lifestyle modifications as well as their effect on patients' quality of life.

Some physicians may adopt a more pragmatic approach toward lifestyle modifications and focus on eliminating only factors that clearly precipitate patients' symptoms.

Table 10–2. Medical Therapeutic Modalities for Noncardiac Chest Pain

<table>
<tr><td colspan="2" align="center">Gastroesophageal Reflux</td></tr>
<tr><td colspan="2">Proton-pump inhibitors</td></tr>
<tr><td>   Omeprazole (Prilosec)</td><td>20 mg p.o. BID</td></tr>
<tr><td>   Rabeprazole (Aciphex)</td><td>20 mg p.o. BID</td></tr>
<tr><td>   Pantoprazole (Protonix)</td><td>40 mg p.o. BID</td></tr>
<tr><td>   Lansoprazole (Prevacid)</td><td>30 mg p.o. BID</td></tr>
<tr><td>   Esomeprazole (Nexium)</td><td>40 mg p.o. BID</td></tr>
<tr><td colspan="2" align="center">Esophageal Dysmotility</td></tr>
<tr><td>Isosorbide dinitrate (Isordil)</td><td>10 mg–20 mg p.o. BID-TID</td></tr>
<tr><td>Diltiazem (Cardizem)</td><td>60 mg–90 mg p.o. QID</td></tr>
<tr><td>Nifedipine (Adalate/Procardia)</td><td>10 mg–30 mg p.o. TID</td></tr>
<tr><td colspan="2" align="center">Visceral Hypersensitivity</td></tr>
<tr><td colspan="2">Tricyclics (commonly used)</td></tr>
<tr><td>   Nortriptyline (Aventyl/Pamelor)</td><td>50 mg p.o. QHS</td></tr>
<tr><td>   Amitriptyline (Elavil/Endep)</td><td></td></tr>
<tr><td>   Doxepin (Sinequan)</td><td></td></tr>
<tr><td>Trazodone (Desyrel)</td><td>100 mg–150 mg p.o. QD</td></tr>
<tr><td>Sertraline (Zoloft)</td><td>50 mg–200 mg p.o. QD</td></tr>
</table>

Histamine-2 Receptor Antagonists (H2RAs)

Cimetidine, ranitidine, nizatidine, and famotidine are the oldest and the most widespread preparations that were used to treat GERD throughout the 1970s and 1980s. Their introduction in the 1970s marked a new era in the treatment of acid-related disorders including GERD.

This class of drugs reduces gastric acid secretion by competitive inhibition of the histamine receptor on the parietal cells. H_2RAs reduce pepsin secretion by an unknown mechanism and reduce gastric acid volume as well.[5] H_2RAs are effective in controlling basal acid secretion but are less effective in suppressing postprandial acid secretion. Although standard doses have been proven to be effective in controlling symptoms and healing of mild to moderate erosive esophagitis, in more severe forms of erosive esophagitis (Los Angeles grades C and D), nonerosive reflux disease, or Barrett's esophagus, H_2RAs are significantly less effective. Kahrilas et al[6] demonstrated that high-dose ranitidine (300 mg bid) failed to improve typical GERD symptoms in more than 50% of patients who experienced persistent heartburn symptoms after 6 weeks of treatment with standard dose ranitidine (150 mg bid).

The efficacy of H_2-receptor antagonists in patients with GERD-related NCCP has been shown to range from 42 to 52%[7] in several published therapeutic studies. DeMeester et al[8] demonstrated that cimetidine (unknown dose) and antacids are effective in only 42% of the patients with GERD-related NCCP who were followed for a period of 2 to 3 years. These results are not surprising as H_2RAs have a limited acid suppressive effect. Additionally, tolerance to H_2RAs generally develops within 2 weeks of repeated administration, resulting in a decline in the acid suppression efficacy.[9] The phenomenon of tolerance to H_2RAs can be explained by the production of a gastrin-induced histamine, which is released by enterochromaffinlike cells (ECLs) in the stomach. Gastrin level is increased in response to elevation in gastric pH, and the histamine that is subsequently produced overpowers the H_2RAs effect on the parietal cells.[10]

Adverse effects of H_2RAs include headache, giddiness, dizziness, fatigue, constipation, diarrhea, and, rarely, impotence.[11]

The role of H_2RAs in the acute and maintenance therapy of GERD has been significantly decreased since the introduction of proton-pump inhibitors (PPIs). Although there are no studies comparing a PPI to an H_2RA in treating GERD-related NCCP, the widely accepted assumption is that H_2RAs will perform poorly in symptoms control as has been repeatedly demonstrated in GERD studies. However, unlike PPIs, H_2RAs are able to provide rapid relief of heartburn that has already developed in patients with GERD, making this class of drugs a preferred on-demand therapeutic modality in GERD. A similar fast effect on acid-induced chest pain has yet to be demonstrated.

Proton-Pump Inhibitors (PPIs)

The introduction of PPIs has revolutionized the treatment of acid-related disorders, and they are currently considered to be the best therapeutic option for all forms of GERD.

The first PPI in the United States, omeprazole, was introduced in 1989, followed by lansoprazole, rabeprazole, pantoprazole, and esomeprazole.

Proton-pump inhibitors are substituted benzimidazole derivatives, which inhibit the proton pump (H+/K+ ATPase) in the parietal cells of the stomach. The proton pump is the final common pathway for gastric acid secretion where hydrogen ions are exchanged with potassium ions. PPIs irreversibly bind to a sulfhydryl group on the proton pump and prevent secretion of acid into the gastric lumen.[12] These compounds control both basal and food-stimulated gastric acid secretion and produce a more profound and longer lasting acid suppression effect than H_2RAs. PPIs are considered the most successful antireflux class of drugs, due to their unsurpassed antisecretory effect resulting in the highest proportion of patients reporting symptom resolution and experiencing complete mucosal healing.[5] The main impact of PPIs has been on erosive esophagitis, complications of GERD, Barrett's esophagus, and atypical/extraesophageal manifestations of GERD.

In an open-label trial, 23 patients with NCCP, who underwent treatment with omeprazole 40 mg at bedtime over a period of 6 weeks, demonstrated a significant reduction in symptom score as compared to baseline.[13] Complete resolution or symptom improvement was seen in 17% and 30% of patients, respectively.

Results of pH testing performed prior to commencement of treatment were not predictive of symptom response.

Achem et al[14] evaluated the effect of omeprazole 20 mg given twice daily over a period of 8 weeks in patients with GERD-related NCCP. In this double-blind, placebo-controlled trial, omeprazole was significantly better than placebo in controlling chest pain symptoms. Although data regarding the efficacy of other PPIs in NCCP are not available, it is highly likely that all PPIs will demonstrate a similar symptom response rate.[15] In general, GERD-related NCCP patients require twice the standard dose of a PPI over a minimum period of 2 months for optimal symptom response. As with other atypical/extraesophageal manifestations of GERD, lag time to symptom resolution may extend to 3 and even 6 months.

Proton-pump inhibitors cause less drug interactions than H_2RAs. Although omeprazole has been shown to interact with diazepam, phenytoin, and warfarin, the clinical significance of such interaction seems to be negligible. Lansoprazole may cause a small decrease in theophylline concentration. However, pantoprazole and rabeprazole appear to be free of these interactions.[16] Tolerance to proton-pump inhibitors has not been reported. As PPIs act at the final step of acid secretion, they effectively block all available mechanisms that promote acid secretion.[10]

Surgical Treatment

Antireflux surgery is an alternative strategy to long-term medical therapy for patients with GERD. Nissen fundoplication is the most commonly performed antireflux operation in patients with symptomatic GERD. The procedure consists of a 360° wrap of the gastric fundus around the distal esophagus, which results in augmentation of the LES basal pressure and a decrease in the rate of transient lower esophageal sphincter relaxations (TLESR). Presently, fundoplication is commonly performed laparoscopically, which is less costly, has less postoperative morbidity, and requires a shorter hospital stay in comparison with open surgery. Postoperatively, however, dysphagia appears to be more common in patients who undergo laparoscopic versus open Nissen fundoplication. Number and severity of postoperative complications closely correlate with the expertise of the surgeon. Common side effects include persistent dysphagia, "gas-bloat" syndrome, inability to vomit, vagal nerve injury, and diarrhea.

Generally, positive response to medical therapy is the best predictor of successful surgical outcome.

The effectiveness of antireflux surgery in GERD-related NCCP is unclear. Several studies demonstrated a positive effect of laparoscopic fundoplication on chest pain in patients with GERD-related NCCP. Patti et al[17] reported that 85% of patients with GERD-related NCCP reported improvement in chest pain symptoms after laparoscopic fundoplication. Farrell et al[18] showed improvement in chest pain and symptom resolution in 90% and 50% of NCCP patients respectively, who underwent antireflux surgery. In contrast, So et al[19] reported that relief of atypical GERD symptoms including chest pain was less satisfactory than relief of typical GERD symptoms, such as heartburn. In their study, 35 consecutive patients underwent laparoscopic fundoplication for atypical GERD symptoms. Patients completed a symptom questionnaire before the operation and 3 and 12 months after the operation. Heartburn was relieved in 93% of the patients, whereas only 48% reported relief of chest pain symptoms. However, results of surgical studies in subjects with atypical/extraesophageal manifestations of GERD are difficult to interpret, because they commonly include a highly selected group of patients.

Endoscopic Treatment

Several endoscopic techniques have been introduced recently for the treatment of GERD. These techniques include endoscopic suturing, radiofrequency ablation, and injection of biocompatible substances. Application of these techniques in GERD remains within the realm of well-designed studies, and their place in the treatment of GERD-related NCCP is presently unknown.

Non-GERD-Related NCCP

The treatment of patients with non-GERD-related NCCP is less rewarding than that of patients with GERD-related NCCP. Whereas altered esophageal pain perception has been demonstrated in all patients with non-GERD-related NCCP, the underlying mechanism responsible for the development of visceral hyperalgesia remains poorly understood. An important development was the recognition that NCCP patients with spastic esophageal motor disorders (except achalasia), as documented by esophageal manometry, are more likely to respond to pain modulators than muscle relaxants. This realization finally brought an end to an era of multiple repeated, failed attempts to treat non-GERD-related NCCP with muscle relaxants.

Esophageal Dysmotility–Pharmacologic Treatment

Traditional pharmacologic options for patients with esophageal motility disorders include nitrates, calcium-channel blockers, and anticholinergic agents (see Table 10–2).[20] In patients with nutcracker esophagus, antireflux medications should be considered before prescribing smooth-muscle relaxants. However, a recently published therapeutic trial (double-blind and placebo-controlled) in NCCP patients with documented nutcracker esophagus demonstrated that lansoprazole 30 mg given twice daily for 8 weeks was not more effective than placebo in relieving chest pain in patients with nutcracker esophagus.[21,22]

Nitrates

Nitroglycerin and long-acting nitrate agents have been shown to cause relaxation of gastrointestinal smooth muscle by stimulating cyclic GMP-dependent pathways. Their effectiveness in patients with esophageal motor disorders was already reported in the medical literature a half a century ago.[23] During the 1970s, several open-label studies reported that nitrates improve symptoms and esophageal manometric patterns in patients with chest pain and esophageal dysmotility. Most investigators noted symptomatic improvement in patients with diffuse esophageal spasm (DES) accompanied by normalization of the motility pattern on esophageal manometry.[24,25] Swamy[26] demonstrated long-term manometric and clinical efficacy of long-acting nitrates in 5 patients with DES. Patients remained asymptomatic during a follow-up of 6 months to 4 years. However, other investigators failed to demonstrate similar efficacy in their studies.[27,28]

Overall, studies that evaluated nitrates were limited to fewer than 50 patients. Only about half of the study subjects had a motility abnormality. The remainder also had GERD or just functional chest pain. A placebo-controlled trial with a priori excluded patients with GERD has yet to be performed.

Overall, long-acting nitrates in doses of 10 to 20 mg two to three times daily have been used, as well as short-acting, sublingual nitrates for acute episodes of chest pain in patients with NCCP.

In conclusion, data are inconsistent about the effectiveness of nitrates in the treatment of patients with NCCP and esophageal dysmotility. This is compounded by adverse effects such as flushing, headaches, and hypotension, which may further limit their clinical utility.

Calcium Channel Blockers

Studies in animal models have demonstrated that calcium plays an important role in esophageal muscle contraction. This led to the assessment of the effect of calcium channel blocking agents such as nifedipine and diltiazem on esophageal motility and symptoms in patients with NCCP. However, as with nitrates, the results of the various studies, mostly open label, are conflicting.

Nifedipine in oral dose of 10 to 30 mg three times daily has been shown to decrease the amplitude and duration of esophageal contractions in patients with nutcracker esophagus.[29] Any notable symptomatic improvement seen in pa-

tients with nutcracker esophagus lasted only 2 weeks. After 6 weeks of therapy, nifedipine completely lost its therapeutic efficacy. Similar results were reported by Davies et al[30] in a double-blind, placebo-controlled trial using nifedipine treatment (10 mg–40 mg 3 times daily) in 20 patients with NCCP and DES. In contrast, Nasrallah et al[31] demonstrated good clinical efficacy of nifedipine given in a dose of 10 mg three times daily in 20 patients with various esophageal motility disorders including hypertensive LES, nutcracker esophagus, diffuse esophageal spasm, and vigorous achalasia.

Diltiazem has been studied in doses of 60 to 90 mg four times daily. In two small studies, it has been shown to significantly improve chest pain score more than placebo in patients with nutcracker esophagus.[32,33] However, in 8 patients with DES, diltiazem was not better than placebo in relieving symptoms of chest pain.[34]

Other Muscle Relaxant Agents

Anticholinergic drugs such as atropine, L-hyoscyamine (the active form of atropine), pirenzepine, and cimetropium bromide can all affect esophageal motility. This may result in reduced amplitude of esophageal contractions and lower esophageal sphincter basal pressure.[35-37]

The antispasmodic cimetropium bromide has been shown to be efficacious in 8 NCCP patients with nutcracker esophagus.[37] Hydralazine, a hypertensive drug that directly dilates peripheral vessels, has been shown to improve chest pain and dysphagia as well as to decrease the amplitude and duration of esophageal contractions in 5 patients.[28]

Endoscopic Treatment

Botulinum toxin (Botox) is an extremely potent bacteroid poison, which blocks acetylcholine-mediated neuromuscular transmission and results in muscle relaxation. Repeated injections of botulinum toxin into the lower esophageal sphincter (LES) have been shown to improve dysphagia and chest pain in patients with achalasia.[38,39] The latter has stimulated investigators' interest in also using this compound for the treatment of nonachalasic esophageal spastic disorders.

Botulinum toxin is usually injected with a 5-mm sclerotherapy needle during an upper endoscopy. In an effort to maximize the amount of medication delivered to the LES, endoscopic ultrasonography may be used to guide injections.[40]

Two trials by Miller and colleagues described the effect of botulinum toxin injections on chest pain scores in patients with esophageal spastic motility disorders. The compound was injected into the LES at doses of 80 to 100 U (4–5 circumferential injections of 20 units each). In the first trial,[41] 15 patients were treated with injections, and 29 patients were treated in the second trial.[42] Favorable symptom response was noted in 67 to 72% of patients.

Recently, Storr et al[43] proposed a provocative approach to NCCP with an esophageal spastic motility disorder. Investigators treated 9 patients suffering from DES with botulinum toxin injections at multiple sites along the esophageal wall. The dosing used in this study was 100 U of drug diluted with 10 mL of saline solution and injected endoscopically from the distal esophagus proximally at 1- to 1.5-cm intervals. Eight of the patients reported a favorable symptom response, but repeated injections were required in half of the cases.

In spite of the aforementioned favorable trials, the clinical effects of botulinum toxin disappear after approximately 6 to 7 months post-therapy. Furthermore, injections may cause local scarring and fibrosis, which may affect future surgical approaches if entertained.[44] Botulinum toxin therapy commonly needs to be repeated to achieve longer duration of symptom response, and the long-term adverse effects of this treatment are still unknown.

Surgical Treatment and Pneumatic Balloon Dilation

Several studies reported that patients with DES may progress over time to achalasia, suggesting that the two clinical disorders may overlap pathophysiologically.[41] Consequently, it has been proposed that treatment for achalasia might also be effective in diffuse esophageal spasm. Pneumatic dilation and surgery are well-established therapeutic options for achalasia, and their effect in diffuse esophageal spasm have been evaluated by several studies.

Successful pneumatic dilation for NCCP and dysphagia caused by diffuse esophageal spasm has been reported in the medical literature.[45] Ebert[46] reported 9 cases with diffuse esophageal spasm and lower esophageal sphincter dysfunction, who were treated by pneumatic dilation. Pneumatic dilation resulted in marked improvement in 8 of the 9 patients during an average follow-up of 37.4 months. Irving[47] studied the effect of pneumatic dilation on 20 patients with severe symptomatic diffuse esophageal spasm who did not respond to medical therapy.

Postdilation, symptoms improved in 14 of the 20 patients.

A thoracic longitudinal myotomy has been reported as a treatment for patients with intractable NCCP caused by non-achalasic esophageal motor disorders. Hendersen et al[48] evaluated 34 patients with diffuse esophageal spasm who failed to respond to medical therapy. Of these, 88% demonstrated marked symptom improvement after extended open esophageal myotomy was performed. Ellis et al[49] reported similar results in 42 patients with NCCP and mostly diffuse esophageal spasm. Cuschieri[50] showed partial or complete relief of chest pain scores in 78% of patients with esophageal spastic motor disorders after thoracoscopic long myotomy.

In contrast, Nastos[51] described 8 patients with spastic esophageal motor disorder who underwent long esophageal myotomy. Four of the patients continued to report severe recurrent chest pain and ultimately underwent esophagectomy. Eypasch[52] described 19 patients with diffuse esophageal spasm who suffered from intractable dysphagia and chest pain. Of these, 15 underwent long esophageal myotomy with an antireflux procedure, and 4 patients with multiple previous esophageal myotomies underwent an esophagectomy. After either myotomy or esophagectomy, the overall symptom score improved significantly. It was concluded in this study that esophagectomy with colonic interposition is the procedure of choice in patients with diffuse esophageal spasm who failed to improve after multiple myotomies.

Patti et al[53] reviewed a prospectively collected database of 397 patients with a diagnosis of primary esophageal motor disorder after esophagogram, endoscopy, manometry, and pH testing. There were 305 patients (77%) with achalasia, 49 patients (12%) with diffuse esophageal spasm (DES), 41 patients (10%) with nutcracker esophagus, and 2 patients (1%) with hypertensive lower esophageal sphincter. Two hundred eight patients (52%) underwent a myotomy by either a thoracoscopic or laparoscopic approach. In achalasia and DES, a thoracoscopic or laparoscopic myotomy relieved dysphagia and chest pain in more than 80% of the patients. However, in nutcracker esophagus the results were less predictable, and the operation most often failed to relieve symptoms. The authors concluded that a laparoscopic Heller myotomy is the primary treatment for achalasia, DES, and hypertensive lower esophageal sphincter with poor results in nutcracker esophagus. Consequently, the authors questioned the concept of nutcracker esophagus as the primary cause for NCCP.

In conclusion, the role of long esophagomyotomy for patients with NCCP and esophageal motor disorder remains to be elucidated. In selected patients with documented diffuse esophageal spasm and failure of medical therapy, long esophageal myotomy could be entertained. Esophagectomy on the other hand may rid the patient from the painful organ but commonly at a devastating cost.

Functional Chest Pain of Presumed Esophageal Origin

The main pathophysiologic mechanism of functional chest pain is visceral hyperalgesia, primarily increased mechanoreceptor sensitivity to balloon distension. Consequently, drugs that alter pain pathways and thus serve as visceral analgesics are currently the mainstay of therapy in these patients. The pain modulators have been shown to improve symptoms regardless if esophageal motility is present or absent.

Several classes of antidepressants, octreotide, and theophylline have all been shown to have visceral analgesic effect that can alleviate chest pain symptoms.

Antidepressants

The rationale for using antidepressants in the treatment of patients with NCCP is multifaceted. First, psychological comorbidity such as anxiety, depression, and others are common in patients with NCCP. Furthermore, patients who suffer from a psychological disorder are more likely to perceive low-intensity esophageal stimuli as painful.[54] Second, studies have demonstrated that antidepressants have a visceral analgesic effect.[55] In addition, antidepressants inhibit calcium channels and thus have a direct effect of muscle relaxants.[56]

Tricyclic antidepressants (TCAs) have been used as pain modulators in various pain syndromes (somatic and visceral). It has been observed that the analgesic effect of TCAs is not dependent on their antidepressant qualities. In fact, the exact mechanism of their analgesic effect remains poorly understood. Studies have shown, however, that TCAs have both a central neuromodulatory and peripheral visceral analgesic effect. The central effect of TCAs appears to act separately from the antidepressant mechanism and thus benefits patients even without psychological comorbidity.[57] The peripheral effect of TCAs depends on their variable receptor affinity. Acetylcholine, histamine, and α-adrenergic receptors are all affected by TCAs, and their variable densities in target tissues alter the pain modulatory action of these drugs. Furthermore, among the class of TCAs, different compounds demonstrate variable affinity to different receptors. Consequently, switching to a different TCA, if one has failed, may prove to be helpful.

Intriguing data about the direct myorelaxant effect of TCAs was recently published by Becker et al.[56] The study demonstrated the effect of antidepressants on smooth muscle contractility of rat's aorta and distal colon. The authors concluded that imipramine and possibly sertraline have myorelaxant properties. This is likely due to better calcium channels blocking properties as compared to other TCA compounds.

Nortriptyline and desipramine are secondary amines (metabolites of tertiary amines) that seem to have fewer side effects. The tertiary amines include amitriptyline, imipramine, doxepin, and others[58] (see Table 10–2).

Numerous clinical trials have found favorable effects of TCAs on esophageal pain perception in both healthy subjects and patients with NCCP. Imipramine at 75 mg daily was shown to significantly increase the pain threshold of healthy males during intraesophageal balloon distension as compared to baseline.[59] In a trial by Cannon et al,[60] 60 patients with chest pain and normal coronary angiography were randomized to receive clonidine (0.2 mg daily), imipramine (50 mg nightly), or placebo for a period of 3 weeks. Only the imipramine group demonstrated a significant reduction (52%) in the number of chest pain episodes. Furthermore, this clinical improvement was independent of the cardiac, esophageal, or psychiatric results. Consequently, the authors concluded that imipramine improves chest pain through a visceral analgesic effect.

Long-term effect of TCAs on functional chest pain was reported by Prakash et al[61] In his study, 21 patients with NCCP were treated with low-dose TCAs after incomplete response to antireflux therapy. Initial treatment resulted in moderate symptom reduction (satisfactory) or remission in 17 subjects (81%). In retrospective analysis, the authors found that 75% of these patients continued to benefit from long-term (up to 3 years) treatment with TCAs. However, drop-out rate was high, in part because of the side effects of these agents.

Common side effects of TCAs include dry mouth, drowsiness, urinary retention, orthostatic hypotension, and constipation.[55] TCAs should be administered at bedtime in a low dose (10–25 mg) and then titrated slowly up to a maximal dose of 50 to 75 mg per day.[58] The incremental increase in dosing should be based on symptoms, development of side effects, and alteration in mood.

Trazodone

Trazodone is used as an antidepressant and/or anxiolytic. The drug effect is possibly mediated by central serotonin reuptake inhibition. Trazodone has been evaluated in a double-blind, placebo-controlled trial that assessed patients with NCCP and esophageal dysmotility.[62] In this study, 15 patients who received trazodone in doses of 100 to 150 mg daily for 6 weeks showed a significantly greater global improvement than 14 patients who received placebo. However, esophageal manometric abnormalities remained unchanged despite therapy with trazodone. In another study, Handa et al[63] reported a positive effect of both trazodone and clomipramine (a TCA), in controlling symptoms of NCCP and manometrically documented diffuse esophageal spasm.

Selective Serotonin Reuptake Inhibitors (SSRIs)

The promising results of trials involving antidepressants such as TCAs and trazodone raised the hope that the selective serotonin reuptake inhibitors (SSRIs) might also have a utility in treating non-GERD-related NCCP patients. This was also supported by a study using citalopram 20 mg IV in normal subjects who underwent various mechanical and chemical painful stimuli.[64] The drug markedly reduced perception thresholds for pain as compared to placebo. Unfortunately, the role of SSRIs in treating NCCP patients has been scarcely studied to date. The efficacy, tolerability, and safety of sertraline in patients with NCCP were evaluated in a randomized, placebo-controlled trial.[65] Thirty patients with a negative stress test or normal coronary angiogram were enrolled. Patients with major depression and panic disorders were excluded from the study. Of those enrolled, 15 patients received sertraline in doses of 50 mg daily, adjusted to a maximum of 200 mg, whereas the other 15 received placebo. By using intention-to-treat analysis, the authors demonstrated a significant advantage of sertraline in reducing chest pain score as compared to placebo.

As with the TCAs, the SSRIs analgesic effect appeared to be independent of their mood-altering properties. Further studies are needed using larger patient population and assessing different SSRIs.

Possible adverse effects of SSRIs include mild nausea, loose stools, decreased libido, and delayed orgasm. However, the SSRIs are associated with significantly fewer adverse reactions as compared to TCAs.

Octreotide

This is a synthetic analog of somatostatin that has been shown to increase rectal and sigmoid visceral perception thresholds for pain in IBS patients and healthy subjects.[66,67] It has been postulated that the effect of octreotide is mediated by the activation of somatostatin receptors at the spinal cord and/or supraspinal level.

Johnston et al[68] evaluated the effect of octreotide, 100 µg subcutaneously, on esophageal pain perception in 12 healthy volunteers, using intraesophageal balloon distension. The authors found that octreotide significantly increased perception thresholds for pain as compared to placebo.

Unfortunately, both high cost and lack of oral formulation prevent the utilization of octreotide in clinical practice.

Theophylline

Recently, adenosine has been identified as a mediator of visceral pain.[69] The adenosine receptor antagonist, theophylline, a xanthine derivative, has been shown to inhibit adenosine-induced anginalike chest pain[70] and adenosine-induced pain in other regions of the body.[71] The favorable effect of theophylline on chest pain in patients with functional chest pain has been demonstrated recently.[72] An esophageal balloon distention protocol, using impedance planimetry, was performed in 21 consecutive patients with functional chest pain. Sixteen patients, who were found to have a hypersensitive esophagus (lower perception thresholds for pain), received intravenous theophylline. The dosage of theophylline was adjusted by body weight. Thirty minutes after completion of the theophylline infusion, the balloon distention protocol was repeated. Perception thresholds for pain increased in 12 (75%) of the patents, and 8 of those continued to receive oral theophylline at a dose of 6 mg per kg per day in two divided doses for a period of 3 months. Oral theophylline completely eliminated chest pain in 1 patient and improved symptoms by at least 50% in 6 others. The authors concluded that theophylline ameliorates chest pain in patients with functional chest pain and documented hypersensitive esophagus by blocking adenosine-mediated nociception.

In another study, the same authors showed that theophylline in an oral dose of 200 mg twice daily was more effective than placebo in preventing chest pain in 19 patients with functional chest pain.[73]

Psychiatric Therapy

Studies have consistently demonstrated that many patients with NCCP, particularly those with functional chest pain, suffer from a variety of psychological disorders most notable, depression and anxiety.[74]

Psychological comorbidity may motivate patients to become avid and sometimes relentless healthcare seekers. If not addressed, psychological comorbidity is likely to interfere with the success of any conventional therapeutic approach for

NCCP. Furthermore, human studies have recently demonstrated that anxiety and stress enhance perception of intraesophageal events, either pathologic or physiologic, by modulating the brain-gut axis.[75]

Treatment for psychological comorbidity has been divided into pharmacologic and nonpharmacologic. Regardless, studies evaluating either modality in NCCP are relatively scarce.

Reassurance has been emphasized as an important mode of therapeutic intervention in patients with NCCP.[76] However, patients' symptoms are seldom relieved by reassurance alone, resulting in the need for additional therapeutic modality.[77]

Pharmacologic Intervention

Several anxiolytics have been evaluated for the treatment of NCCP, mostly from the benzodiazepines class of drugs. Recently, Huffman[78] reviewed the role of benzodiazepines in the treatment of patients with chest pain. The authors concluded that these medications may be useful as a therapeutic modality, primarily in patients with chest pain caused by diffuse esophageal spasm, achalasia, nutcracker esophagus, and nonspecific motility disorders.

Alprazolam (Xanax) has shown efficacy at a mean dose of 4.3 mg per day in patients with NCCP and panic disorder.[79] This study revealed that 15 out of 20 patients reported at least 50% reduction in episodes of panic attacks and a corresponding decline in the frequency of chest pain episodes.

Clonazepam in doses of 1 to 4 mg per day was shown to be effective in treatment of 27 patients with NCCP and panic disorder.[80]

Nonpharmacologic Intervention

Psychotherapy may also be helpful in the treatment of patients with NCCP, particularly when accompanied by hypochondriasis, anxiety, or panic disorder.

Several studies have demonstrated that patients with NCCP treated with cognitive-behavioral therapy report significant improvement of quality of life and reduction in chest pain symptoms.[81] Additionally, cognitive-behavioral therapy has been successfully used for the treatment of patients with NCCP without relation to existing panic disorder.[82] The latter study evaluated 31 patients who were treated with cognitive-behavioral therapy. Of those, 15 (48%) patients remained pain free at 12 months of follow-up, as compared to only 4 (13%) of the 33 patients in the control group (without intervention).

Other psychological interventions that have been suggested to work in patients with NCCP include reassurance, education, relaxation techniques, breathing training, and biofeedback.

Biofeedback was assessed in a study that compared this approach to primary care visits only in patients with NCCP.[83] Patients in the biofeedback group demonstrated a significantly lower symptom frequency and severity. However, a large group of patients assigned to the biofeedback arm (52%) did not complete the study.

Hypnotherapy versus supportive therapy were recently compared in a very small trial that included only 28 NCCP patients.[84] The authors demonstrated that patients receiving hypnotherapy reported significant improvement in chest pain, primarily due to reduction in intensity and not frequency, as compared to the control arm. The study, which embarked on a parallel group design, is likely too small to provide any conclusions about the full clinical effect of hypnotherapy in NCCP patients.

Future Treatment

New therapeutic modalities are unlikely to be developed specifically for NCCP. However, successful pain modulators developed for irritable bowel syndrome or functional dyspepsia will most likely also be evaluated in patients with non-GERD-related NCCP, regardless if esophageal dysmotility is present or absent.

Many of the compounds under investigation target peripheral receptors of neurotransmitters that are thought to play an important role in pain perception. Many potential targets are currently under consideration. They include vanilloid receptor ion channels, acid-sensing ion channels, sensory neuron-specific Na+ channels, P2X purinoceptors, cholecystokinin (CCK) receptors, 5-hydroxytryptamine (5-HT) receptors, bradykinin and prostaglandin receptors, glutamate receptors, tachykinin, and calcitonin gene-related peptide receptors as well as peripheral opioid and cannabinoid receptors.[85]

Some of the currently available compounds that are either already clinically approved or under investigation include 5-HT receptors agonists and antagonists (partial $5HT_4$ agonist and $5HT_3$ antagonist), neurokinin receptors (NK1 and NK2) antagonists, N-methyl-D-aspartate (NMDA) receptor antagonist, cholecystokinin-A receptor antagonist, and calcitonin-gene-related peptide (CGRP) antagonist. These are all potential new visceral analgesics that may have an effect on symptoms of patients with non-GERD-related NCCP.

5-Hydroxytryptamine (5-HT) Antagonists and Agonists

Serotonin (5-HT) is a neurotransmitter that is present in the central nervous system, enteric neurons, and extrinsic afferents of the gut. Presently, it is considered to be involved in the processes of visceral perception and motor activity of the gastrointestinal tract (Table 10–3).[86]

Numerous subtypes of 5-HT receptor have been identified in the CNS as well as the gastrointestinal tract (see Table 10–3). Studies in IBS have focused primarily on $5\text{-}HT_3$ receptor antagonists and partial $5\text{-}HT_4$ receptor agonists. The $5\text{-}HT_3$ receptors are present on the enteric and spinal neurons. Alosetron, the first $5\text{-}HT_3$ receptor antagonist on the market, was found to have a visceral analgesic effect in animal models and humans. The drug has been shown to reduce discomfort and pain in female patients with IBS.[87,88] Alosetron was removed from the market because of adverse effects and is currently available for patients with severe IBS only. However a new $5\text{-}HT_3$ antagonist will be introduced into the market shortly. Ondansetron, a $5\text{-}HT_3$ antagonist used as an antiemetic, has been shown to increase esophageal perception thresholds for pain in patients with NCCP.[89] However, the wide usage of this drug in non-GERD-related NCCP is hampered by cost and the availability of efficacious and cheaper pain modulators (such as TCAs and trazodone).

The $5\text{-}HT_4$ receptor agonists such as prucalopride and tegaserod improve general gastrointestinal propulsion.[90]

Table 10–3. Overview of 5-HT Receptors and Those Suitable for Use in Human Drugs

Subtype	Selective Agonist	Selective Antagonist	Nonselective Agonist	Nonselective Antagonist
1A			Buspirone	
1B	Sumatriptan			
1D	Sumatriptan			
1F				
2A		Ketanserin		Mianserin
2B				
2C				
3		Odansetron		
		Granisetron		
		Alosetron		
		Tropisetron		
4	Tegaserod		Cisapride	
	Prucalopride		Renzapride	

Adapted from Tack and Sarnelli (2005)[86]

Tegaserod has been suggested to have a pain modulatory effect but is currently approved for the treatment of women with constipation-predominant IBS. Studies with tegaserod in patients with non-GERD-related NCCP are warranted.[91]

Nonserotonergic Agents

Peripheral opioid receptors are of immense interest because they may offer visceral analgesic effect without crossing the blood-brain barrier and thus affecting the CNS. The peripherally acting kappa opioid agonist fedotozine may have a beneficial effect in patients suffering from non-GERD-related NCCP. Fedoto-

zine, which acts as a peripheral antinociceptive compound, has been shown to reduce perception of intracolonic balloon distensions in IBS patients.[92]

Tachykinin antagonists are spinal afferents that play a role in visceral nociception expressed tachykinins. Tachykinins are a family of biologically active peptides that include substance P, neurokinins A and B, as well as neuropeptide K. Tachykinin antagonists may confer a visceral analgesic effect that can be used in non-GERD-related NCCP patients. Neurokinin (NK)-1, NK-2, and NK-3 receptor antagonists were mostly evaluated in preclinical trials.

Cholecystokinin-A receptor antagonists: Loxiglumide, a cholecystokinin receptor antagonist, is currently under clinical evaluation for treatment of various functional bowel disorders. The drug acts by accelerating gastric emptying and colonic transit, thereby increasing the number of bowel movements in patients with chronic constipation. It has also been suggested that cholecystokinin-A receptor antagonists alter visceral pain.[93] However, studies in NCCP are still unavailable.

Acid pump antagonists: This class of drugs inhibits the proton pump at the potassium channel preventing the exchange of potassium and hydrogen ions needed for acid secretion. The acid pump antagonists are characterized by rapid onset of action, predictable dose response effect, profound acid suppression, and lack of dependency on meals. This class of drugs may play an important role in the treatment of GERD-related NCCP and potentially as a better therapeutic test.

Summary

NCCP is a heterogeneous disorder with different underlying mechanisms responsible for patients' symptoms. Although treatment of patients with NCCP remains a challenge, the availability of highly potent antireflux medications in the last decade has markedly improved our ability to treat patients with GERD-related NCCP. In these patients, proton-pump inhibitors, at least twice daily for acute therapy and in many for maintenance therapy, are needed to control symptoms. In patients with non-GERD-related NCCP, pain modulators such as tricyclic antidepressants, trazodone, and SSRIs are currently the cornerstone of treatment,

regardless if esophageal dysmotility is present or not. Presently, concurrent diagnosis of esophageal dysmotility (except achalasia) should not influence the treatment plan, and all patients should be prescribed a visceral analgesic.

Psychological comorbidity is very common in patients with NCCP and should not be overlooked. Pharmacologic or nonpharmacologic approaches have been used with varied success. Further studies are needed to determine the best psychological approach to NCCP patients. Future therapy for NCCP will include visceral analgesic compounds as well as new and more potent antireflux medications.

References

1. Richter JE. Chest pain and gastroesophageal reflux disease. *J Clin Gastroenterol.* 2000;30(3 suppl):S39–S41.
2. Fass R, Fennerty MB, Johnson C, Camargo L, Sampliner RE. Correlation of ambulatory 24-hour esophageal pH monitoring results with symptom improvement in patients with noncardiac chest pain due to gastroesophageal reflux disease. *J Clin Gastroenterol.* 1999;28(1):36–39.
3. Fass R, Bautista J, Janarthanan S. Treatment of gastroesophageal reflux disease. *Clin Cornerstone.* 2003;5(4):18–29.
4. Kitchin LI, Castell DO. Rationale and efficacy of conservative therapy for gastroesophageal reflux disease. *Arch Intern Med.* 1991;151(3):448–454.
5. Fass R, Hixson LJ, Ciccolo ML, Gordon P, Hunter G, Rappaport W. Contemporary medical therapy for gastroesophageal reflux disease. *Am Fam Physician.* 1997; 55(1):205–212.
6. Kahrilas PJ, Fennerty MB, Joelsson B. High-versus standard-dose ranitidine for control of heartburn in poorly respon-

sive acid reflux disease: a prospective, controlled trial. *Am J Gastroenterol.* 1999;94(1):92–97.

7. Fang J, Bjorkman D. A critical approach to noncardiac chest pain: pathophysiology, diagnosis, and treatment. *Am J Gastroenterol.* 2001;96(4):958–968.

8. DeMeester TR, O'Sullivan GC, Bermudez G, Midell AI, Cimochowski GE, O'Drobinak J. Esophageal function in patients with angina-type chest pain and normal coronary angiograms. *Ann Surg.* 1982;196(4):488–498.

9. Jones R, Bytzer P. Review article: acid suppression in the management of gastro-oesophageal reflux disease-an appraisal of treatment options in primary care. *Aliment Pharmacol Ther.* 2001;15(6):75–77.

10. Sandvik AK, Brenna E, Waldum HL. Review article: the pharmacological inhibition of gastric acid secretion—tolerance and rebound. *Aliment Pharmacol Ther.* 1997;11(6):1013–1018.

11. Piper DW. A comparative overview of the adverse effect of antiulcer drugs. *Drug Saf.* 1995;12(2):120–138.

12. Pisegna JR. Pharmacology of acid suppression in the hospital setting: focus on proton pump inhibition. *Crit Care Med.* 2002;30(6 suppl):S356–S361.

13. Chambers J, Cooke R, Anggiansah A, Owen W. Effect of omeprazole in patients with chest pain and normal coronary anatomy: initial experience. *Int J Cardiol.* 1998;65(1):51–55.

14. Achem SR, Kolts BE, MacMath T, et al. Effects of omeprazole versus placebo in treatment of noncardiac chest pain and gastroesophageal reflux. *Dig Dis Sci.* 1997;42(10):2138–2145.

15. Fass R. Chest pain of esophageal origin. *Curr Opin Gastroenterol.* 2002;18:464–470.

16. Horn J. The proton-pump inhibitors: similarities and differences. *Clin Ther.* 2000;22(3):266–280.

17. Patti MG, Molena D, Fisichella PM, Perretta S, Way LW. Gastroesophageal reflux disease (GERD) and chest pain. Results of laparoscopic antireflux surgery. *Surg Endosc.* 2002;16(4):563–566.

18. Farrell TM, Richardson WS, Trus TL, Smith CD, Hunter JG. Response of atypical symptoms of gastro-oesophageal reflux to antireflux surgery. *Br J Surg.* 2001;88(12):1649–1652.

19. So JB, Zeitels SM, Rattner DW. Outcomes of atypical symptoms attributed to gastro-esophageal reflux treated by laparoscopic fundoplication. *Surgery.* 1998;124(1):28–32.

20. Achem SR, Kolts BE. Current medical therapy for esophageal motility disorders. *Am J Med.* 1992;92(5A):98S–105S.

21. Achem SR, Kolts BE, Wears R, Burton L, Richter JE. Chest pain associated with nutcracker esophagus: a preliminary study of the role of gastroesophageal reflux. *Am J Gastroenterol.* 1993;88(2):187–192.

22. Borjesson M, P R, Mannheimer C, Pilhall M. Nutcracker oesophagus: a double-blind, placebo-controlled, cross-over study of the effects of lansoprazole. *Aliment Pharmacol Ther.* 2003;18(11–12):1129–1135.

23. Schmidt HW. Diffuse spasm of lower half of the esophagus. *Dig Dis.* 1939;6:693–700.

24. Orlando RC, Bozymski EM. Clinical and manometric effects of nitroglycerin in diffuse esophageal spasm. *N Engl J Med.* 1973;289(1):23–25.

25. Millaire A, Ducloux G, Marquand A, Vaksmann G. Nitroglycerin and angina with angiographically normal corona vessels. Clinical effects and effects on esophageal motility. *Arch Mal Coeur Vaiss.* 1989;82(1):63–68.

26. Swamy N. Esophageal spasm: clinical and manometric response to nitroglycerine and long acting nitrites. *Gastroenterology.* 1977;72(1):23–27.

27. Kikendall JW, Mellow MH. Effect of sublingual nitroglycerin and long-acting nitrate preparations on esophageal motility. *Gastroenterology.* 1980;79(4):703–706.

28. Mellow MH. Effect of isosorbide and hydralazine in painful primary esophageal

motility disorders. *Gastroenterology.* 1982;83(2):364-370.

29. Richter JE, Dalton CB, Buice RG, Castell DO. Nifedipine: a potent inhibitor of contractions in the body of the human esophagus. Studies in healthy volunteers and patients with the nutcracker esophagus. *Gastroenterology.* 1985;89(3):549-554.

30. Davies HA, Lewis MJ, Rhodes J, Henderson AH. Trial of nifedipine for prevention of oesophageal spasm. *Digestion.* 1987; 36(2):81-83.

31. Nasrallah SM, Tommaso CL, Singleton RT, Backhaus EA. Primary esophageal motor disorders: clinical response to nifedipine. *South Med J.* 1985;78(3):312-315.

32. Richter JE, Spurling TJ, Cordova CM, Castell DO. Effects of oral calcium blocker, diltiazem, on esophageal contractions. Studies in volunteers and patients with nutcracker esophagus. *Dig Dis Sci.* 1984;29(7):649-656.

33. Cattau EL, Jr. , Castell DO, Johnson DA, et al. Diltiazem therapy for symptoms associated with nutcracker esophagus. *Am J Gastroenterol.* 1991;86(3):272-276.

34. Drenth JP, Bos LP, Engels LG. Efficacy of diltiazem in the treatment of diffuse oesophageal spasm. *Aliment Pharmacol Ther.* 1990;4(4):411-416.

35. Phaosawasdi K, Malmud LS, Tolin RD, Stelzer F, Applegate G, Fisher RS. Cholinergic effects on esophageal transit and clearance. *Gastroenterology.* 1981;81(5): 915-920.

36. Jaup BH, Abrahamsson H, Virtanen R, Iisalo E. Effect of pirenzepine compared with atropine and L-hyoscyamine on esophageal peristaltic activity in humans. *Scand J Gastroenterol.* 1982;17(2): 233-239.

37. Bassoti G, Gaburri M, Imbimbo BP, et al. Manometric evaluation of cimetropium bromide activity in patients with the nutcracker oesophagus. *Scand J Gastroenterol.* 1988;23(9):1079-1084.

38. Pasricha PJ, Ravich WJ, Kalloo AN. Botulinum toxin for achalasia. *Lancet.* 1993; 341(8839):244-245.

39. Cuilliere C, Ducrotte P, Zerbib F, et al. Achalasia: outcome of patients treated with intrasphincteric injection of botulinum toxin. *Gut.* 1997;41(1):87-92.

40. Miller LS, Schiano TD. The use of high frequency endoscopic ultrasonography probes in the evaluation of achalasia. *Gastrointest Endosc Clin North Am.* 1995;5(3):635-647.

41. Miller LS, Parkman HP, Schiano TD, et al. Treatment of symptomatic nonachalasia esophageal motor disorders with botulinum toxin injection at the lower esophageal sphincter. *Dig Dis Sci.* 1996; 41(10):2025-2031.

42. Miller LS, Pullela S, Parkman HP, et al. Treatment of chest pain in patients with noncardiac, nonreflux, nonachalasia spastic esophageal motor disorders using botulinum toxin injection into the gastroesophageal junction. *Am J Gastroenterol.* 2002;97(7):1640-1646.

43. Storr M, Allescher HD, Rosch T, Born P, Weigert N, Classen M. Treatment of symptomatic diffuse esophageal spasm by endoscopic injection of botulinum toxin: a prospective study with long term follow-up. *Gastrointest Endosc.* 2001; 54(6):18A.

44. Bhutani MS. Gastrointestinal uses of botulinum toxin. *Am J Gastroenterol.* 1997; 92(6):929-933.

45. Patterson DR. Diffuse esophageal spasm in patients with undiagnosed chest pain. *J Clin Gastroenterol.* 1982;4(5):415-417.

46. Ebert EC, Ouyang A, Wright SH, Cohen S, Lipshutz WH. Pneumatic dilatation in patients with symptomatic diffuse esophageal spasm and lower esophageal sphincter dysfunction. *Dig Dis Sci.* 1983;28(6): 481-485.

47. Irving JD, Owen WJ, Linsell J, McCullagh M, Keightley A, Anggiansah A. Management of diffuse esophageal spasm with balloon dilatation. *Gastrointest Radiol.* 1992;17(3):189-192.

48. Henderson RD, D R, Marryatt G. Extended esophageal myotomy and short total fundoplication hernia repair in dif-

fuse esophageal spasm: five-year review of 34 patients. *Ann Thorac Surg.* 1987; 43(1):25–31.

49. Ellis FH, Jr. Esophagomyotomy for non-cardiac chest pain resulting from diffuse esophageal spasm and related disorders. *Am J Med.* 1992;92(5A):129S–131S.

50. Cuschieri A. Endoscopic oesophageal myotomy for specific motility disorders and non-cardiac chest pain. *Endosc Surg Allied Technol.* 1993;1(5–6):280–287.

51. Nastos D, Chen LQ, Ferraro P, Taillefer R, Duranceau AC. Long myotomy with anti-reflux repair for esophageal spastic disorders. *J Gastrointest Surg.* 2002;6(5): 713–722.

52. Eypasch EP, DeMeester TR, Klingman RR, Stein HJ. Physiologic assessment and surgical management of diffuse esophageal spasm. *J Thorac Cardiovasc Surg.* 1992; 104(4):859–868.

53. Patti M, Gorodner M, Galvani C, et al. Spectrum of esophageal motility disorders: implications for diagnosis and treatment. *Arch Surg.* 2005;140:442–449.

54. Trimble KC, Pryde A, Heading RC. Lowered oesophageal sensory thresholds in patients with symptomatic but not excess gastro-oesophageal reflux: evidence for a spectrum of visceral sensitivity in GORD. *Gut.* 1995;37(1):7–12.

55. Egbunike IG, Chaffee BJ. Antidepressants in the management of chronic pain syndromes. *Pharmacotherapy.* 1990;10(4): 262–270.

56. Becker B, Morel N, Vanbellinghen AM, Lebrun P. Blockade of calcium entry in smooth muscle cells by the antidepressant imipramine. *Biochem Pharmacol.* 2004;68(5):833–842.

57. Camilleri M. Management of the irritable bowel syndrome. *Gastroenterology.* 2001; 120(3):652–668.

58. Clouse RE. Psychotropic medications for the treatment of functional gastrointestinal disorders. *Clin Perspect Gastroenterol.* 1999;2:348–356.

59. Peghini PL, Katz PO, Castell DO. Imipramine decreases oesophageal pain per-ception in human male volunteers. *Gut.* 1998;42(6):807–813.

60. Cannon RO, 3rd, Quyyumi AA, Mincemoyer R, et al. Imipramine in patients with chest pain despite normal coronary angiograms. *N Engl J Med.* 1994;330(20): 1411–1417.

61. Prakash C, Clouse RE. Long-term outcome from tricyclic antidepressant treatment of functional chest pain. *Dig Dis Sci.* 1999;44(12):2373–2379.

62. Clouse RE, Lustman PJ, Eckert TC, Ferney DM, Griffith LS. Low-dose trazodone for symptomatic patients with esophageal contraction abnormalities. A double-blind, placebo-controlled trial. *Gastroenterology.* 1987;92(4):1027–1036.

63. Handa M, Mine K, Yamamoto H, et al. Antidepressant treatment of patients with diffuse esophageal spasm: a psychosomatic approach. *J Clin Gastroenterol.* 1999;28(3):228–232.

64. Broekaert D, Fischler B, Sifrim D, Janssens J, Tack J. Influence of citalopram, a selective serotonin reuptake inhibitor, on oesophageal hypersensitivity: a double-blind, placebo-controlled study. *Aliment Pharmacol Ther.* 2006;23(3):365–370.

65. Varia I, Logue E, O'connor C, et al. Randomized trial of sertraline in patients with unexplained chest pain of noncardiac origin. *Am Heart J.* 2000;140(3): 367–372.

66. Bradette M, Delvaux M, Staumont G, Fioramonti J, Bueno L, Frexinos J. Octreotide increases thresholds of colonic visceral perception in IBS patients without modifying muscle tone. *Dig Dis Sci.* 1994;39(6):1171–1178.

67. Schwetz I, Naliboff B, Munakata J, et al. Anti-hyperalgesic effect of octreotide in patients with irritable bowel syndrome. *Aliment Pharmacol Ther.* 2004;19(1): 123–131.

68. Johnston BT, Shils J, Leite LP, Castell DO. Effects of octreotide on esophageal visceral perception and cerebral evoked potentials induced by balloon distension. *Am J Gastroenterol.* 1999;94(1):65–70.

69. Bueno L, Fioramonti J, Delvaux M, Frexinos J. Mediators and pharmacology of visceral sensitivity: from basic to clinical investigations. *Gastroenterol.* 1997;112(5): 1714-1743.

70. Crea F, Pupita G, Galassi AR, et al. Role of adenosine in pathogenesis of anginal pain. *Circulation.* 1990;81(1):164-172.

71. Pappagallo M, Gaspardone A, Tomai F, Iamele M, Crea F, Gioffre PA. Analgesic effect of bamiphylline on pain induced by intradermal injection of adenosine. *Pain.* 1993;53(2):199-204.

72. Rao SS, Mudipalli RS, Mujica V, Utech CL, Zhao X, Conklin JL. An open-label trial of theophylline for functional chest pain. *Dig Dis Sci.* 2002;47(12):2763-2768.

73. Mudipalli RS, Utech CL, Kempf J, Rao SS. A double blind, placebo controlled crossover study of oral theophylline in functional chest pain [abstract]. *Gastroenterology.* 2003;124(suppl 1):A122.

74. Esler JL, Bock BC. Psychological treatments for noncardiac chest pain: recommendations for a new approach. *J Psychosom Res.* 2004;56(3):263-269.

75. Fass R, Malagon I, Naliboff BD, Pulliam G, Peleg N, Mayer EA. Effect of psychologically induced stress on symptom perception and autonomic nervous system response of patients (PTS) with erosive esophagitis (EE) and non-erosive reflux disease (NERD) [abstract]. *Gastroenterology.* 2000;118(4):A637, 3250.

76. Ågård A, Bentley B, Herlitz J. Experiences and concerns among patients being treated for atypical chest pain. *Eur J Intern Med.* 2005;16:339-344.

77. Clouse R, Carney R. The psychological profile of non-cardiac chest pain patients. *Eur J Gastroenterol.* 1995;7(12):1160-1165.

78. Huffman JC, Stern TA. The use of benzodiazepines in the treatment of chest pain: a review of the literature. *J Emerg Med.* 2003;25(4):427-437.

79. Beitman BD, Basha IM, Trombka LH, et al. Pharmacotherapeutic treatment of panic disorder in patients presenting with chest pain. *J Fam Pract.* 1989;28(2): 177-180.

80. Wulsin LR, Maddock R, Beitman B, Dawaher R, Wells VE. Clonazepam treatment of panic disorder in patients with recurrent chest pain and normal coronary arteries. *Int J Psychiatry Med.* 1999;29(1):97-105.

81. Klimes I, Mayou RA, Pearce MJ, Coles L, Fagg JR. Psychological treatment for atypical non-cardiac chest pain: a controlled evaluation. *Psychol Med.* 1990;20(3): 605-611.

82. van Peski-Oosterbaan AS, Spinhoven P, van Rood Y, van der Does JW, Bruschke AV, Rooijmans HG. Cognitive-behavioral therapy for noncardiac chest pain: a randomized trial. *Am J Med.* 1999;106(4): 424-429.

83. Ryan M, Gervirtz R. Biofeedback-based psychophysiological treatment in a primary care setting: an initial feasibility study. *Appl Psychophysiol Biofeedback.* 2004;29(2):79-93.

84. Jones H, Cooper P, Miller V, Brooks N, Whorwell P. Treatment of non-cardiac chest pain: a controlled trial of hypnotherapy. *Gut.* 2006;55(10):1403-1408.

85. Holzer P. Gastrointestinal afferents as targets of novel drugs for the treatment of functional bowel disorders and visceral pain [review]. *Eur J Pharmacol.* 2001;429(1-3):177-193.

86. Tack J, Sarnelli G. Serotonergic modulation of visceral sensation: upper gastrointestinal tract. *Gut.* 2002;51(suppl 1): i77-i80.

87. Bardhan KD, Bodemar G, Geldof H, et al. A double-blind, randomized, placebo-controlled dose-ranging study to evaluate the efficacy of alosetron in the treatment of irritable bowel syndrome. *Aliment Pharmacol Ther.* 2000;14(1):23-34.

88. Talley NJ, Van Zanten SV, Saez LR, et al. A dose-ranging, placebo-controlled, randomized trial of alosetron in patients with functional dyspepsia. *Aliment Pharmacol Ther.* 2001;15(4):525-537.

89. Stark M, Maher K, Gupta P. Visceral afferent blockade with ondasetron increases

nociceptive thresholds in patients with non cardiac chest pain [abstract]. *Am J Gastroenterol.* 1991;18:A129.

90. Bouras EP, Camilleri M, Burton DD, McKinzie S. Selective stimulation of colonic transit by the benzofuran 5HT4 agonist, prucalopride, in healthy humans. *Gut.* 1999;44(5):682–686.

91. Fass R, Tougas G. Functional heartburn: the stimulus, the pain, and the brain. *Gut.* 2002;51(6):885–892.

92. Delvaux M, Louvel D, Lagier E, Scherrer B, Abitbol JL, Frexinos J. The kappa agonist fedotozine relieves hypersensitivity to colonic distention in patients with irritable bowel syndrome. *Gastroenterology.* 1999;116(1):38–45.

93. Scarpignato C, Pelosini I. Management of irritable bowel syndrome: novel approaches to the pharmacology of gut motility. *Can J Gastroenterol.* 1999; 13(suppl A):50A–65A.

CHAPTER 11

Economics (Direct and Indirect Costs) of Noncardiac Chest Pain

Guy D. Eslick

Introduction

The economics of noncardiac chest pain (NCCP), in terms of direct or indirect costs, remains largely speculative.[1] There are few if any data concerning the direct health care costs associated with noncardiac chest pain; however, there are a couple of studies that have determined some of the indirect costs related to noncardiac chest pain.[2]

Noncardiac chest pain places a substantial drain on hospital resources; the condition accounts for approximately 2 to 5% of all emergency presentations and is one of the most frequent causes of hospital admissions in the western world.[3] Community education regarding the importance of recognizing chest pain symptoms and the early presentation to hospital to reduce morbidity and mortality has been the focus of a number of cardiovascular organizations around the world. In spite of this, over the last decade, most hospitals have observed a stabilization or decline in the number of presentations with acute myocardial infarction, while there has been a proportionately greater increase in admissions with noncardiac chest pain (defined as chest pain not due to underlying detectable ischemic heart disease) (Fig 11-1).

Direct Costs

Direct costs are the costs of the materials and labor that go directly into production of goods or services, such as labor, materials, and equipment. The emerging increase in chest pain presentations to hospital emergency departments would also suggest that the levels of health care utilization and the costs (both direct and indirect) associated with noncardiac chest pain are going to increase.

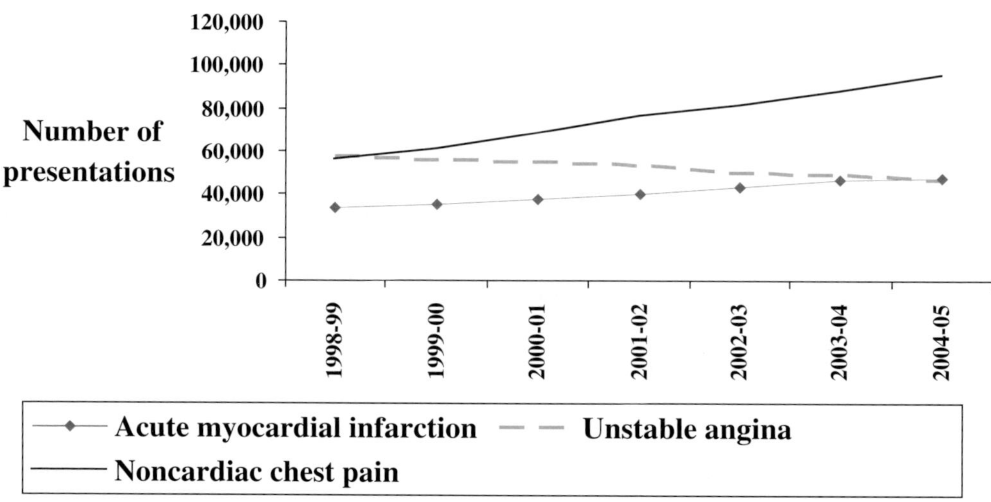

Fig 11–1. Changes over time in noncardiac chest pain, unstable angina, and acute myocardial infarction rates for Australia. (From the Australian Institute of Health and Welfare [AIWH], National Hospital Morbidity Database.)

It should be noted that those studies assessing cost-effectiveness have focused on treatment rather than diagnostic testing.[4-6] There have been a few cost-effectiveness analysis studies conducted assessing the efficacy of empirical therapy for noncardiac chest pain.[4-6] The first study was conducted by Fass and colleagues,[5] who wanted to estimate the potential cost savings of using omeprazole as a diagnostic test in patients with NCCP ($n = 39$) compared with conventional diagnostic evaluations. A cost-effectiveness analysis revealed that the omeprazole saves $573 per patient evaluated and resulted in a 59% reduction in the number of diagnostic procedures undertaken. Another study using decision/cost-effectiveness analysis also assessed noncardiac chest pain patients who were treated with omeprazole and compared it with the diagnostic tests used. The study reported that using omeprazole for treating noncardiac chest pain patients (followed if necessary by ambulatory pH monitoring, then manometry,

and then endoscopy), was the most effective and least expensive option and resulted in an 11% improvement in diagnostic accuracy, and a 43% reduction in the use of invasive diagnostic tests, which led to an average cost savings of $454 per patient, compared with the strategy of commencing with endoscopy, then pH monitoring, and then manometry.[6] Borzecki et al[5] conducted another decision/cost-effectiveness analysis to assess the empirical treatment in patients with noncardiac chest pain using antisecretory agents compared with investigation. Costs associated with initial investigation were $2,187 per case compared with $849 for the empirical treatment (which remained dominant for just over 12 months). There are major limitations to these "decision/cost-effectiveness analysis" studies; most only use modeling-based assumptions and probabilities from the literature, which may not reflect the current practice or the "real world" in terms of clinical options and noncardiac chest pain outcomes in the long term.

There have been reports that noninvasive testing is cost-effective for patients who present with chest pain.[7-10] Kuntz et al[7] compared several interventions including, no testing, exercise ECG, exercise echocardiography, exercise SPECT, and coronary angiography using a cost-effectiveness analysis and sensitivity analysis. The study reported that both exercise ECG and echocardiography were cost-effective for patients with mild to moderate risk of coronary heart disease. However, it must be noted that this study did not specifically report on patients with noncardiac chest pain and the diagnostic procedures referred to in the study were used to determine coronary artery disease (ie, exercise electrocardiogram, coronary angiography). Another cardiac chest pain study compared the costs of an emergency department-based accelerated diagnostic protocol, based on tests that detect acute myocardial infarction during its early stages, against hospitalization in patients with chest pain.[8] The primary outcomes measured were the total cost of treatment and the length of stay (LOS). This study suggested that using the accelerated diagnostic protocol saved $567 in total hospital costs per patient treated and also reduced hopitalization rates, length of stay, and total costs for low-risk patients with chest pain. This study did not differentiate patients into cardiac and noncardiac chest pain groups.

Indirect Costs

Studies assessing the indirect economic costs of noncardiac chest pain are rare. This is remarkable considering the high population prevalence and "suspected" high economic burden of noncardiac chest pain.[1,11,12] Chest pain has long been recognized as an occupational disability, being ranked as one of the top four reasons for absenteeism from work.[11,12]

Work Absenteeism

Until recently, the majority of studies have been on patients with cardiac chest pain.[13-16] One such study, a large (*n* = 2,250) multicenter study of coronary angioplasty patients reported that the occurrence of chest pain during follow-up was an important predictor of return to work, no matter what the outcome of the angioplasty. In addition, 77% of patients with chest pain were working at follow-up, compared to 90% of patients without chest pain. Furthermore, several studies of other potential noncardiac chest pain-related conditions, such as gastroesophageal reflux disease (GERD), imply that the impact of absenteeism is substantial.[17-21] Frank et al[17] found that lost productivity at work due to reflux symptoms accounted for at least 4% of work-related absenteeism and this increased to 11% if a comorbid motility disorder was present. Another study reported that GERD was accountable for a substantial decrease in work productivity (41%), which represented a 3% loss in total productivity.[18] A Swedish study of GERD patients with mild-to-moderate reflux symptoms were assessed using a validated, self-report productivity scale (The Work Productivity and Activity Instrument), and found that as symptom severity increased from mild to severe there was also an increase in reduced work productivity from 16 to 32%. At present there is only one study that assesses absenteeism and noncardiac chest pain.[2] This hospital-based study of individuals presenting with chest pain

(n = 212), compared cardiac and noncardiac chest pain patients. Overall, the prevalence of missing work or school in the previous 12 months because of chest pain was 28% (95% CI: 22-35%) for all chest pain, 25% (95% CI: 15-38%) for cardiac chest pain patients, and 29% (95% CI: 21-38%) for noncardiac chest pain patients. The average number of days absent for all chest pain was 22 days in the previous 12 months (range: 1-240 days), for cardiac chest pain patients it was 22 days (range: 2-56 days), and for noncardiac chest pain patients it was 25 days (range: 1-240 days). There was no significant difference in days absent between cardiac and noncardiac chest pain patients. The findings from this study suggest that absenteeism among chest pain patients is common with the frequency of absenteeism higher among those with noncardiac chest pain compared to cardiac chest pain patients. Future studies are required to assess the effect of noncardiac chest pain on work productivity and to replicate these findings in other populations.

Summary

For the large part, the real costs associated with noncardiac chest pain remain hidden (Fig 11-2). There is a dearth of studies on the economics of noncardiac chest pain, making this a fertile area for future research. Due to the lack of studies, the true economic impact and burden of noncardiac chest pain remain speculative at best. Based on the increasing epidemiology, long natural history, and extensive testing associated with these patients one can assume that both

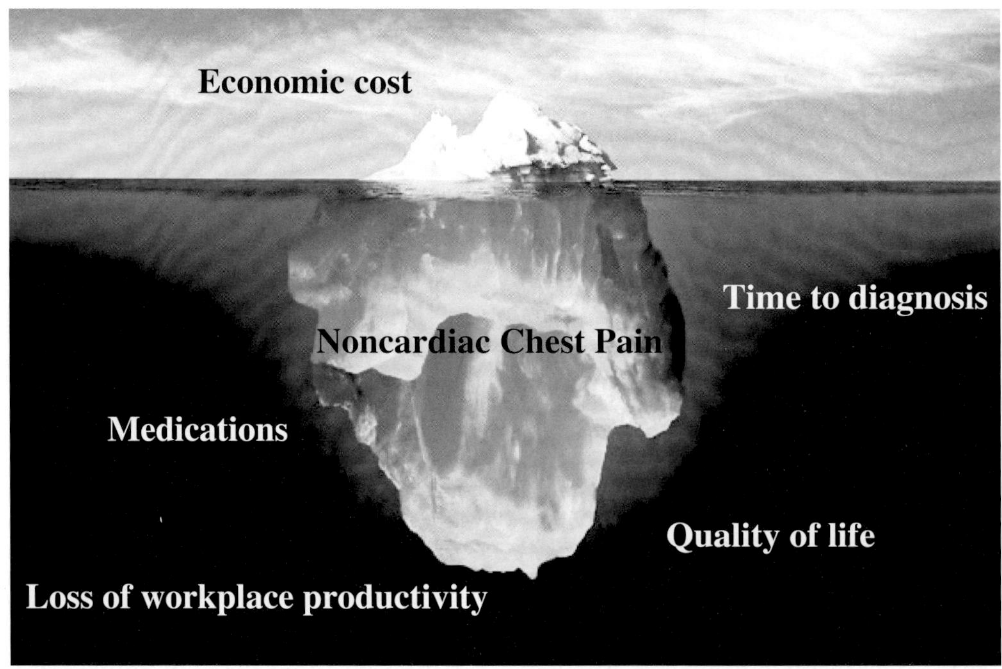

Fig 11–2. What lies beneath? The real costs of noncardiac chest pain.

the direct and indirect costs associated with noncardiac chest pain are substantial; however, these require quantification.

References

1. Eslick GD, Coulshed DS, Talley NJ. The burden of illness of non-cardiac chest pain. *Aliment Pharmacol Ther*. 2002; 16:1217-1223.
2. Eslick GD, Talley NJ. Non-cardiac chest pain: predictors of health care seeking, the types of health care professional consulted, work absenteeism, and interruption of daily activities. *Aliment Pharmacol Ther*. 2004;20:909-915.
3. Eslick GD, Talley NJ. Non-cardiac chest pain: squeezing the life out of the Australian healthcare system? *Med J Aust*. 2000;173:233-234.
4. Borzecki AM, Pedrosa MC, Prashker MJ. Should noncardiac chest pain be treated empirically? *Arch Intern Med*. 2000;160: 844-852.
5. Fass R, Fennerty MB, Ofman JJ, et al. The clinical and economic value of short course of omeprazole in patients with noncardiac chest pain. *Gastroenterology*. 1998;115:42-49.
6. Ofman JJ, Gralnek IM, Udani J, Fennerty MB, Fass R. The cost-effectiveness of the omeprazole test in patients with noncardiac chest pain. *Am J Med*. 1999;107: 219-227.
7. Kuntz KM, Fleischmann KE, Hunink MGM, Douglas PS. Cost-effectiveness of diagnostic strategies for patients with chest pain. *Ann Intern Med*. 1999;130: 709-718.
8. Roberts RR, Zalenski RJ, Mensah EK, et al. Costs of an emergency department-based accelerated diagnostic protocol vs hospitalization in patients with chest pain. *JAMA*. 1997;278:1670-1676.
9. Shebuski RJ. Utility of point-of-care diagnostic testing in patients with chest pain and suspected acute myocardial infarction. *Curr Opin Pharmacol*. 2002;2:160-164.
10. Marini G, Boni G, Barreca M, et al. Radionuclide gastroesophageal motor studies. *J Nuclear Med*. 2004;45:1004-1028.
11. Mayou R. The patient with angina: symptoms and disability. *Postgraduate Medical J*. 1973;49:250-254.
12. Achem SR, DeVault KR. Recent developments in chest pain of undetermined origin. *Curr Gastroenterol Reports*. 2000;2: 201-209.
13. Beitman BD, Mukerji V, Lamberti JW, et al. Panic disorder in patients with chest pain and angiographically normal coronary arteries. *Am J Med*. 1989;63:1399-1403.
14. Engblom E, Korpilahti K, Hamalainen H, Ronnemaa T, Puukka P. Quality of life and return to work 5 years after coronary artery bypass surgery: long-term results of cardiac rehabilitation. *J Cardiopulmonary Rehabil*. 1997;17:29-36.
15. Holmes DR Jr, Van Raden MJ, Reeder GS, et al. Return to work after coronary angioplasty: a report from the national heart, lung, and blood Institute percutaneous transluminal coronary angioplasty registry. *Am J Cardiol*. 1984;53:48C-51C.
16. Lisspers J, Sundin O, Hofman-Bang C, et al. Behavioral effects of a comprehensive, multifactorial program for lifestyle change after percutaneous transluminal coronary angioplasty: a prospective, randomised, controlled study. *J Psychosomatic Res*. 1999;46:143-154.
17. Frank L, Klineman L, Ganoczy D, et al. Upper gastrointestinal symptoms in North America: prevalence and relationship to healthcare utilization and quality of life. *Dig Dis Sci*. 2000;45:809-818.
18. Henke CJ, Levin TR, Henning JM, Potter LP. Work loss costs due to peptic ulcer disease and gastroesophageal reflux disease in a health maintenance organization. *Amer J Gastroenterol*. 2000;95: 788-792.
19. Bloom BS, Jayadevappa R, Wahl P, Cacciamanni J. Time trends in cost of caring for people with gastroesophageal reflux

disease. *Am J Gastroenterol.* 2001; 96(suppl 1):S64–S69.

20. Wahlqvist P, Carlsson J, Stalhammar NO, Wiklund I. Validity of a work productivity and activity impairment questionnaire for patients with symptoms of gastro-esophageal reflux disease (WPAI-GERD): results from a cross-sectional study. *Value in Health.* 2002;5:106–113.

21. Levin TR, Schmittdiel JA, Kunz K, et al. Costs of acid-related disorders to a health maintenance organization. *Am J Med.* 1997;103;520–528.

CHAPTER 12

Quality of Life

Guy D. Eslick

Introduction

It is assumed that noncardiac chest pain (NCCP) impacts on the quality of life of sufferers; however, there are very few studies assessing quality of life (QoL) among individuals with noncardiac chest pain. The majority of these are hospital-based studies with only one population-based study.

Hospital-Based Studies

Five studies have been hospital-based in design.[1-4] A Spanish study assessed a newly developed quality of life instrument (specifically designed for patients with cardiac syndrome X) among patients ($n = 90$) with cardiac syndrome X (defined as "the presence of typical, ischaemia like, chest pain, and ECG changes during pain in patients with normal coronary angiograms")[5] and found that quality of life was significantly impaired in patients with cardiac syndrome X.[1] A major limitation of this study was the lack of a comparison group with which to compare the quality of life instrument and scores. Moreover, the classification of cardiac syndrome X remains a contentious issue, and thus it may or may not be a noncardiac condition. Another study, conducted by Wong and colleagues[4] compared 78 noncardiac chest pain patients and 20 healthy controls undergoing endoscopy; all subjects completed the SF-36 quality of life questionnaire.[4] Across all SF-36 domains, noncardiac chest pain patients reported lower scores than healthy controls. There were three domains (physical functioning, role physical, and general health perceptions) where there were significant differences between the two groups.

An Australian hospital-based study was recently conducted; some of these data have been reported[6]; however, the data presented here have not been published previously.[3] The study consisted of 212 patients who presented to a tertiary hospital emergency department with acute chest pain and were assessed according to a standard diagnostic protocol that included an exercise (ECG) stress test and completed the Chest Pain Questionnaire (CPQ). One hundred and twenty-six had noncardiac chest pain, with 71 classified as having cardiac chest pain. When comparing the individual subscale scores of those with cardiac chest pain versus those with noncardiac chest pain, those with cardiac chest pain had lower scores, indicating greater impaired quality of life on the SF-36. The score differences were less than 5 points for the subscales role physical, vitality, and mental health indicating clinically relevant changes (Table 12–1). However, univariate analysis found that there was only one statistically significant quality of life subscale (mental health index) that had a lower score among the noncardiac chest pain subjects compared to those who had a cardiac cause for their chest pain.

A recent German study found that among a sample of consecutive patients ($n = 37$) with anginalike chest pain and normal coronary angiograms that high priority psychiatric and orthopedic evaluation along with esomeprazole administration might confirm the causes of noncardiac chest pain.[7] The patients underwent testing for psychiatric, musculoskeletal disorders, and GERD, and also completed the SCL-90 (for anxiety, depression, panic, and somatization), along with the SF-36 and the Seattle Angina Questionnaire. The authors reported that the recognition of psychiatric disorders is extremely important among this group of patients due to the substantially reduced quality of life and ineffective passive coping mechanisms (praying, hoping,

catastrophizing).[7] A limitation of this study was the selection of noncardiac chest pain patients that were recruited; all had undergone coronary angiography. However, in clinical practice the majority of noncardiac chest pain patients rarely have a coronary angiogram.

The final study was conducted to determine whether childhood and current adversities were more widespread in patients with noncardiac chest pain and the associated health-related quality of life.[2] The study subjects consisted of consecutive patients attending gastroenterology and cardiology clinics who were interviewed for childhood experience of care and abuse and life events and difficulties schedules. Quality of life was assessed using the SF-36 at the initial clinic visit and again 6 months later. There were 133 total patients, only 40 of whom reported noncardiac chest pain; the remaining had other conditions including functional dyspepsia ($n = 43$), gastroesophageal reflux disease (GERD) ($n = 29$), and ischemic heart disease ($n = 21$). The authors report that there was no significant difference in childhood adversity, social stress, a lack of a close confidant, and levels of psychological distress between the diagnostic groups. However, a multiple logistic regression analysis found that childhood adversity was an independent predictor for patients with noncardiac chest pain and functional dyspepsia, but not for gastroesophageal reflux disease or ischemic heart disease. This study suggested that childhood adversity was common among these select groups and was associated directly with poor outcome only in patients with noncardiac chest pain and functional dyspepsia.

These five hospital-based studies have evaluated different groups of patients

Table 12–1. Quality of Life (SF-36) Scores for Hospital-Based Patients with Noncardiac and Cardiac Chest Pain

		Noncardiac Chest Pain	Cardiac Chest Pain	*P*-value
SF-36 Physical Functioning (0–100)	Mean	64.24	59.33	0.26
	SD	26.27	30.00	
SF-36 Role Physical (0–100)	Mean	33.68	25.67	0.12
	SD	34.51	32.63	
SF-36 Pain Index (0–100)	Mean	59.11	55.55	0.40
	SD	27.59	29.88	
SF-36 General Health Perceptions (0–100)	Mean	57.28	55.23	0.56
	SD	23.09	22.54	
SF-36 Vitality (0–100)	Mean	45.37	51.39	0.09
	SD	25.08	21.61	
SF-36 Social Functioning (0–100)	Mean	61.24	56.53	0.24
	SD	25.34	28.77	
SF-36 Role Emotional (0–100)	Mean	65.19	62.96	0.73
	SD	41.40	42.80	
SF-36 Mental Health Index (0–100)	Mean	68.66	74.14	0.04*
	SD	18.14	17.23	

SD = Standard Deviation; *p* <0.05.

and control groups, providing interesting findings with respect to quality of life. Overall, the findings suggest that those with noncardiac chest pain have a significantly worse quality of life than normal healthy controls. Recent research suggests that those with noncardiac chest pain do not differ in their quality of life compared to those with a cardiac cause for their chest pain, except for mental health which was significantly worse for those with noncardiac chest pain. Moreover, one of the recent studies not only reported a substantially reduced quality of life among those with noncardiac chest pain, but also found that these patients had ineffective passive coping mechanisms.

Population-Based Studies

Up to now there has been only one study assessing the impact of quality of life on individuals with noncardiac chest pain in the community.[8] The authors found that when comparing the individual subscale scores in those with no chest pain and those with noncardiac chest pain, there were lower scores in the noncardiac chest pain individuals, indicating impaired quality of life on the SF-36. The score differences were all less than 5 points, indicating clinically relevant changes except for the subscale physical functioning (Table 12-2). Among those with severe noncardiac chest pain and those with mild

Table 12–2. Quality of Life (SF-36) Scores Comparing Those with Nil Pain, All, Mild, and Severe Noncardiac Chest Pain in the Community

		Nil Pain	All Noncardiac Chest Pain	Mild Noncardiac Chest Pain	p-value (nil vs mild)	Severe Noncardiac Chest Pain	*P*-value (nil vs severe)
SF-36 Physical Functioning (0–100)	Mean	83.28	81.63	83.72	0.9	69.70	0.003*
	SD	21.62	22.92	21.57		26.82	
SF-36 Role Physical (0–100)	Mean	82.11	74.04	76.39	0.09	60.00	0.001*
	SD	31.72	36.76	35.43		41.83	
SF-36 Pain Index (0–100)	Mean	78.01	70.08	71.71	<0.001*	60.75	0.001*
	SD	24.91	24.09	23.36		26.43	
SF-36 General Health Perceptions (0–100)	Mean	75.48	67.68	68.87	<0.001*	60.98	<0.001*
	SD	19.10	19.96	18.98		24.03	
SF-36 Vitality (0–100)	Mean	62.05	53.26	54.46	<0.001*	46.41	<0.001*
	SD	19.98	21.28	21.20		20.76	
SF-36 Social Functioning (0–100)	Mean	85.44	78.37	79.44	<0.001*	72.26	<0.001*
	SD	22.93	24.26	23.14		29.57	
SF-36 Role Emotional (0–100)	Mean	82.89	73.49	74.81	0.004*	65.55	0.01*
	SD	30.93	36.62	35.52		42.42	
SF-36 Mental Health Index (0–100)	Mean	76.38	69.05	69.82	<0.001*	64.62	0.007*
	SD	17.35	19.20	18.16		24.17	

SD = Standard Deviation; *p <0.05.

Reproduced from *Aliment Pharmacol Ther.* 2003;17:1115-1124, with permission.

noncardiac chest pain there were significant differences between all the mean scores, with worse scores in severe noncardiac chest pain for each individual subscale on the SF-36. These results suggest that increasing severity of noncardiac chest pain leads to a worse quality of life compared to mild symptoms, thus making it an extremely incapacitating condition.

Qualitative Studies

A Swedish group of noncardiac chest pain patients ($n = 20$) has been the subject of two recently published articles aiming to gain a greater understanding of quality of life among noncardiac chest pain patients using qualitative methods.[9,10] The first report aimed to describe patients' experience of noncardiac chest pain and how the pain affected their everyday life.[9] The sample consisted of 19 individuals (58% male) who were admitted to the emergency department with chest pain. The qualitative assessment for each patient included an open-ended unstructured interview. Overall, the patients provided descriptions of their pain experience covering several categories including (a) pain location, (b) pain duration with the subcategories "periodic pain" and "continuous pain," (c) pain intensity, (d) quality of pain with the subcategories "sensory aspects" and "affective aspects." Moreover, the pain experience in terms of everyday life was further divided into the following groups (i) fear and anxiety, (ii) feeling of uncertainty, (iii) feeling of stress, and (iv) loss of strength. The findings from this study suggested that chest pain significantly affected the everyday lives of the participants. The second

report aimed to describe the experience of noncardiac chest pain and its influence on everyday life among males and females.[10] The methodology involved the same subjects as in the first report, along with a qualitative descriptive methodology with interviews. The interviews revealed two areas of focus, which included "descriptions" and "consequences" of chest pain in an individual's daily life. Patients described their chest pain using words such as pressure, cramp, strong, or burning with similar terms used between genders. In terms of the physical, psychological, and social consequences associated with chest pain in daily life, males reported a "fast tempo" in their lives, with stress at work reported by both males and females. The conclusions from this study suggest that males and females had more similarities in terms of both the descriptions and consequences of their chest pain than differences.

Summary

It is clear that noncardiac chest pain has an enormous impact in terms of quality of life among those who suffer with this condition. Currently, although it is known that severity is important and that increasing severity of chest pain symptoms decreases quality of life, the effect in terms of symptom frequency on individuals has not been reported in terms of quality of life. The effects are universal and do not differ between those who present to hospital emergency departments or those who live in the community with noncardiac chest pain. Physicians need to have a greater understanding of the effects of noncardiac chest pain in terms of an individual's "quality of life" when assessing patients and how individuals will differ in terms of pain response, psychological response, and physical response.

References

1. Atienza F, Velasco JA, Brown S, Ridocci F, Kaski JC. Assessment of quality of life in patients with chest pain and normal coronary arteriogram (syndrome X) using a specific questionnaire. *Clin Cardiol.* 1999;22:283–290.
2. Biggs, A-M. Aziz, Q. Tomenson, B. Creed, F. Effect of childhood adversity on health related quality of life in patients with upper abdominal or chest pain. *Gut.* 2004;53:180–186.
3. Eslick GD. (2004). *The Epidemiology of Non-cardiac Chest Pain* [Dissertation]. Department of Medicine, The University of Sydney.
4. Wong WM, Lai KC, Lau CP, et al. Upper gastrointestinal evaluation of Chinese patients with non-cardiac chest pain. *Aliment Pharmacol Ther.* 2002;16:465–471.
5. Kaski JC. *Chest Pain with Normal Coronary Angiograms: Pathogenesis, Diagnosis and Management.* Boston, Mass: Kluwer Academic Publishers; 1999.
6. Eslick GD, Talley NJ. Non-cardiac chest pain: predictors of health care seeking, the types of health care professional consulted, work absenteeism, and interruption of daily activities. *Aliment Pharmacol Ther.* 2004;20:909–915.
7. Husser D, Bollmann A, Kuhne C, Molling J, Klein U. Evaluation of noncardiac chest pain: diagnostic approach, coping strategies and quality of life. *Eur J Pain.* 2006; 10:51–55.
8. Eslick GD, Jones MP, Talley NJ. Non-cardiac chest pain: prevalence, risk factors, impact and consulting—a population-based study. *Aliment Pharmacol Ther.* 2003;17:1115–1124.
9. Jarlock M, Gaston-Johansson F, Danielson E. Living with unexplained chest pain. *J Clin Nursing.* 2005;14:956–964.
10. Fagring AJ, Gaston-Johansson F, Danielson E. Description of unexplained chest pain and its influence on daily life in men and women. *Eur J Cardiovascular Nursing.* 2005;4:337–344.

CHAPTER 13

Prognosis

Guy D. Eslick

Introduction

The natural history of noncardiac chest pain (NCCP) remains largely unknown.[1] Several hospital-based studies have assessed the prospective outcomes of patients with noncardiac chest pain.[2-11] When comparing the results from these studies, it should be noted that not all these studies have classified noncardiac chest pain the same way; there is considerable overlap and inconsistency in the definitions used for noncardiac chest pain. Thus, there are significant differences in study findings.

Early Studies

One of the earliest studies reported was by Wielgosz and colleagues,[3] which consisted of a 1-year morbidity and mortality follow-up of patients (n = 821) with chest pain and normal coronary arteries as determined by coronary angiography.

At follow-up, more than two-thirds of patients (67%) continued to experience chest pain to some extent with 39% reporting less pain, 26% the same pain, and 2% having more severe pain. During the follow-up period only three patients died (0.3%), and all were due to non-ischemic reasons. An 11-year follow-up study conducted in the United Kingdom to assess the psychological morbidity on 46 chest pain patients with normal coronary arteries found that only four patients had died during the course of the study and that the causes of death were stroke, cancer, suicide, and ischemic heart disease.[2] At follow-up, 31 (74%) of the surviving 42 patients reported chest pain in the preceding 6 months and 18 (39%) had chest pain at least once a week. In addition, there have been intermediate term (5-year) follow-up studies of patients with "atypical" chest pain that report more than two-thirds (74%) not only continued to have chest pain for 5 years but that this was associated with impaired functional status and increased health care seeking because of their chest pain.[4,5] Moreover, further studies have also reported similar findings in terms of continued chest pain and impaired functional status.[6-10]

Wilhelmsen et al[11] conducted one of the longest follow-up studies, which consisted of a 16-year follow-up. The study found that both cardiac and noncardiac mortality was high among males aged between 51 to 59 years ($n = 6,488$) with chest pain who did not have angina pectoris. Overall, the relative risk of death related to ischemic heart disease among males with noncardiac chest pain was 2.8 (95% CI: 2.20-3.50). However, this study was limited by the fact that it only included older males; hence, the results of this study are not generalizable as there is no comparison with females or males from younger age groups.

Conventionally, patients with noncardiac chest pain are assumed to have an outstanding prognosis; however, specific studies assessing the natural history of noncardiac chest pain are uncommon. A large number of patients report the persistence of chest pain symptoms, impaired functional status, and the chronic use of drugs (cardiac, gastrointestinal, psychiatric) with frequent admissions to the hospital including medical procedures such as cardiac catheterizations.[12]

Recent Studies

A recent prospective cohort study of noncardiac chest pain patients has aimed to determine the natural history of non-cardiac chest pain and related symptoms over a 4-year period.[13] The sample consisted of patients who presented to the Nepean Hospital Emergency Department in Sydney with acute chest pain. At initial presentation, patients who elected to undergo further diagnostic tests were assessed according to a standard protocol. All patients were asked to fill out the valid Chest Pain Questionnaire (CPQ),[14,15] including those who did not wish to undergo further diagnostic procedures. At 2 and 4 years after first presentation, the patients were sent another CPQ to complete and return that measured symptoms, risk factors, psychological distress, quality of life, and general demographics. At baseline there were 126 (60%) non-cardiac chest pain patients and 71 cardiac patients. Chest pain continued to be reported in the majority of individuals (>65%) at follow-up. Over the 2-year period noncardiac chest pain disappeared among 10% ($n = 9/88$), but remained present in the remaining 90% ($n = 79$). In comparison, 69% ($n = 28/41$) of the cardiac chest pain patients continued to have chest pain at the 2-year follow-up (noncardiac chest pain vs cardiac chest pain: $p<0.001$). At the 4-year follow-up 71% ($n = 45/64$) and 81% (23/27) continued to have noncardiac chest pain and cardiac chest pain, respectively ($p <0.001$). The mortality rate among the entire cohort over the 4-year study was 9% (17/197). The cardiac mortality rate for patients initially diagnosed with cardiac chest pain was 11% (8/71); compared with 5.5% (7/126) ($p = 0.16$) among patients initially diagnosed with noncardiac chest pain who subsequently died from a cardiac cause. The outcomes in terms of mortality did not significantly differ between cardiac and noncardiac chest pain patients. Moreover, the majority in both groups experienced continued chest pain during the follow-up period. Consequently noncardiac chest pain does not always confer an excellent intermediate-term prognosis.

Summary

The data regarding the prognosis of non-cardiac chest pain are conflicting with some studies suggesting an excellent prognosis whereas others have found outcomes associated with noncardiac chest pain patients to be similar to those with acute coronary syndromes. A few possible reasons for the differences found may relate to the accuracy of the initial "chest pain" diagnosis, the definition of noncardiac chest pain used in some of these studies, the selection procedures used for recruiting patients, and the outcomes selected. Patients with noncardiac chest pain need to be reassured that their condition is not life threatening (after a full cardiac examination and assessment), and physicians who are unable to provide patients with a "diagnosis" or treatment should not be surprised to see these patients more frequently. Referral to other specialities including psychological medicine should be made if an organic cause for a patient's chest pain cannot be discovered.

References

1. Eslick GD, Coulshed DS, Talley NJ. Diagnosis and treatment of noncardiac chest pain. *Nat Clin Pract Gastroenterol Hepatol*. 2005;2:463–472.

2. Potts SG, Bass CM. Psychological morbidity in patients with chest pain and normal or near-normal coronary arteries: a long-term follow-up study. *Psychol Med*. 1995;25:339–347.

3. Wielgosz AT, Fletcher RH, McCants CB, et al. Unimproved chest pain in patients with minimal or no coronary disease a behavioral phenomenon. *Am Heart J*. 1984;108:67–72.

4. Roll M, Kollind M, Theorell T. Five-year follow-up of young adults visiting an emergency unit because of atypical chest pain. *J Intern Med*. 1992;231:59–65.

5. Tew R, Guthrie EA, Creed FH, Cotter L, Kisley S, Tomenson B. A long-term follow-up study of patients with ischemic heart disease versus patients with nonspecific chest pain. *J Psychosom Res*. 1995;39:977–985.

6. Kisely S, Guthrie E, Creed F, Tew R. Predictors of mortality and morbidity following admission with chest pain. *J Roy Coll Phys Lond*. 1997;31:177–183.

7. Launbjerg J. The long-term prognosis of patients with acute chest pain, but without myocardial infarction. *Danish Med Bull*. 1997;44:365–379.

8. Gurevitz O, Jonas M, Boyko V, Rabinowitz B, Reicher-Reiss H. Clinical profile and long-term prognosis of women <50 years of age referred for coronary angiography for evaluation of chest pain. *Am J Cardiol*. 2000;85:806–809.

9. Ward BW, Wu WC, Richter JE, Hackshaw BT, Castell DO. Long-term follow-up of symptomatic status of patients with non-cardiac chest pain: is diagnosis of esophageal etiology helpful? *Am J Gastroenterol*. 1987;82:215–218.

10. Karlson BW, Wiklund I, Bengtson A, Herlitz J. Prognosis, severity of symptoms, and aspects of well-being among patients in whom myocardial infarction was ruled out. *Clin Cardiol*. 1994;17:427–431.

11. Wilhelmsen L, Rosengren A, Hagman M, Lappas G. "Nonspecific" chest pain associated with high long-term mortality: Results from the primary prevention study in Goteborg, Sweden. *Clin Cardiol*. 1998;21:477–482.

12. Hallani H, Eslick GD, Cox M, Ma Wyatt J, Lee CH. Chest pain: ? cause. *Lancet*. 2004;363:452.

13. Eslick GD, Talley NJ. The natural history of non-cardiac chest pain (NCCP): a four-year prospective cohort study. *Gastroenterology*. 2004a;126(suppl 2):A-310.

14. Eslick GD, Talley NJ. The development and validation of the Chest Pain Questionnaire (CPQ) for non-cardiac chest pain (NCCP). *Gastroenterology*. 2004b; 126(suppl 2):A-309.

15. Eslick GD, Jones MP, Talley NJ. Non-cardiac chest pain: prevalence, risk factors, impact and consulting—a population-based study. *Alimentary Pharmacol Ther*. 2003;17:1115–1124.

CHAPTER 14

Noncardiac Chest Pain— The Future

Ronnie Fass

The area of NCCP will continue to evolve in the next decade. Whereas interest in the disease has somewhat diminished and the number of groups actively involved in research in this field has decreased over the years, clinicians and patients alike will remain highly interested in NCCP because of its high prevalence in the general population.

The epidemiology and economic impact of the disease have not been fully elucidated. Studies are needed to further characterize patients with NCCP, particularly, ethnic and gender predilection, age distribution, and health-seeking behavior. Surprisingly, several recent studies have demonstrated that primary care physicians treat more than three-quarters of patients diagnosed with NCCP and elect not to refer them to a gastroenterologist for further evaluation.[1] Furthermore, half of the patients diagnosed with NCCP are treated by their cardiologist; and of those referred, approximately 50% are sent back to their primary care physician rather than to a gastroenterologist.[2] These findings suggest that most NCCP patients are treated by specialties that are not fully exposed to the current NCCP literature. In fact, both studies clearly demonstrated that the primary care physicians and cardiologists do not follow current practices in NCCP. Consequently, publications and educational programs targeting the primary care physicians and cardiologists would help to bring these physicians up to date.

The introduction of the Bravo™ capsule has already helped to elucidate the relationship between patients' chest pain reports and acid reflux events. Specifically, longer duration of pH recording provides a better opportunity to capture chest pain symptoms and associate them with acid reflux events.[3]

The future introduction of the acid pump antagonists (APAs), also called potassium channel blockers, may dramatically improve the sensitivity of the current PPI test in diagnosing GERD-related

NCCP. This class of drugs possesses a more rapid onset of action, independent of meal stimulation than presently available PPIs, a more predictable dose-response effect, and better antisecretory properties. The APAs will require extensive evaluation, but these agents may play an important role in GERD-related NCCP as a diagnostic tool ("the APA test") or as an improved short- and long-term treatment for GERD-related NCCP.

The role of nonacidic reflux as the underlying mechanism for chest pain will be evaluated, using the new multichannel intraluminal impedance. Although the clinical value of this technique remains to be fully elucidated, enthusiasm about its value in GERD is quite high. The latter is likely to serve as the impetus for exploratory studies in GERD-related NCCP.

Research into the underlying mechanisms that result in the development of NCCP may ultimately lead to novel therapeutic modalities. Future research will continue to focus on mechanisms for pain in NCCP patients, primarily the role of central and peripheral sensitization in enhancing perception of intraesophageal stimuli. Alosetron, a 5-hydroxytryptamine (5HT) type 3 antagonist, which was previously available for the treatment of female patients with diarrhea-predominant irritable bowel syndrome, raised the hope for a therapeutic potential in patients with NCCP.[4] This class of drugs appears to have a pain-modulatory effect, probably by altering the initiation, transmission, or processing of extrinsic sensory information from the gastrointestinal tract. Tegaserod, a partial 5HT type 4 agonist, has recently been shown to modulate pain perception in patients with functional heartburn undergoing balloon distention protocol. However,

the role of tegaserod in NCCP has yet to be determined.

Phosphorylation of N-methyl-D-aspartate (NMDA) receptors expressed by dorsal horn neurons leads to central sensitization via increase in their excitability and receptive field size.[5] Potentially, this central sensitization may be prevented or even reversed by antagonism of NMDA receptors within the spinal cord. However, it is important to note that central nervous system mechanisms that mediate visceral hyperalgesia are sensitive to both NMDA-receptor blockers and non-NMDA-receptor antagonists.[6]

Potential targets that are currently under consideration include vanilloid receptor ion channels, acid-sensing ion channels, sensory neuron-specific Na+ channels, P2X purinoceptors, cholecystokinin (CCK) receptors, bradykinin and prostaglandin receptors, glutamate receptors, tachykinin, and calcitonin gene-related peptide receptors as well as peripheral opioid and cannabinoid receptors.[7] The peripheral opioid receptor agonists are of high interest because they may offer visceral analgesic effect without crossing the blood-brain barrier and thus affecting the CNS.

Spinal afferents, which may play a role in visceral nociception, express tachykinins, (a family of biologically active peptides) that includes substance P, neurokinins A and B, and neuropeptide K.) Tachykinin antagonists may confer a visceral analgesic effect that can be used in non-GERD-related NCCP patients. Neurokinin (NK)-1, NK-2, and NK-3 receptor antagonists have only been evaluated in preclinical trials. Cholecystokinin receptor antagonists, like loxiglumide, may alter visceral pain perception.[8] However, studies in NCCP are still unavailable.

Another important area that is likely to attract future attention is complementary and alternative therapeutic modalities that can interfere with the mind and body axis. Interestingly, despite the increase in public interest in these modalities, thus far, very few studies have assessed their role in NCCP patients.

The role of endoscopic therapy in patients with GERD-related NCCP has been scarcely studied. Although most endoscopic techniques have lost their appeal due to potential severe or even fatal complications, questionable long-term efficacy, and improvement of only subjective clinical endpoints, new prototypes are presently under evaluation and are likely to reach the market within a year or two. If the therapeutic efficacy of the "second generation endoscopic therapy for GERD" will be superior to the currently available endoscopic techniques, it is highly likely that special patient populations, like those with NCCP, will be evaluated as well. Lastly, antireflux surgery will remain limited to a carefully selected group of patients with NCCP. This trend is unlikely to change in the short term.

References

1. Wong W-M, Risner-Adler S, Beeler J, et al. Attitudes and referral patterns of primary care physicians when evaluating subjects with noncardiac chest pain—A survey. *Dig Dis Sci.* 2005;50:656–661.
2. Wong W-M, Risner-Adler S, Beeler J, et al. The role of the cardiologist—A national survey. *J Clin Gastroenterol* (in press).
3. Prakash C, Clouse R. Wireless pH monitoring in patients with non-cardiac chest pain. *Am J Gastroenterol.* 2006;101(3): 446–452.
4. Burbige EJ. Use of a 5-HT$_3$ antagonist in a patient with noncardiac chest pain [abstract]. *Gastroenterology.* 2001;96(9): S183, #579.
5. Sarkar S, Aziz Q, Woolf CJ, et al. Contribution of central sensitisation to the development of non-cardiac chest pain. *Lancet.* 2000;356:1154–1159.
6. Cervero F. Visceral hyperalgesia revised [commentary]. *Lancet.* 2000;356:1127–1128.
7. Holzer P. Gastrointestinal afferents as targets of novel drugs for the treatment of functional bowel disorders and visceral pain (review). *Eur J Pharmacol.* 2001; 429(1–3):177–193.
8. Scarpignato C, Pelosini I. Management of irritable bowel syndrome: novel approaches to the pharmacology of gut motility. *Can J Gastroenterol.* 1999; 13(suppl A):50A–65A.

Index

T

Tachykinin antagonists, 150
TCA (tricyclic antidepressants), 44, 136,
        137, 138, 145, 151
Tegaserod, 149–150, 174
Tetracyclines, 50
Texidor's twinge, 44
Theophylline, 137, 140, 147
Thermal stimulation testing, 65–66
Thoracentesis, 49
Thyroid dysfunction, 43
Tietze, Alexander (1864–1927), 42
Tietze's syndrome, 42, 43
Transient receptor potential vanilloid type 1
        (TRPV1), 66
Trazodone, 136, 138, 146, 151
Treatment. *See also* Medications;
        Psychological comorbidity
    aerobic exercise, 44
    biofeedback, 148
    botulinum toxin injection, 143
    calcium-channel blockers, 142
    cognitive behavioral therapy (CBT), 44,
        148
    costochondritis, 43
    endoscopic, 141, 143
    esophageal dysmotility, 138, 141–144
    esophagectomy, 144
    fibromyalgia, 44
    functional pain (presumed esophageal),
        antidepressants, 145–146
        nonpharmacologic, 148–149
        octreotide, 147
        psychiatric therapy, 147–148
        SSRI (selective serotonin reuptake
            inhibitors), 146–147
        theophylline, 147
        trazodone, 146
    future, 149–151
    GERD,
        H_2RA (histamine$_2$-receptor antagonists,
            139
        lifestyle modifications, 137
        PPI, 139–140
    H_2RA (histamine$_2$-receptor antagonists),
        versus PPI, 139, 140
    hypnotherapy, 148–149

    intercostal nerve block, 42
    nitrates, 141–142
    non-GERD NCCP, 141
    overview, 135–137, 151
    PPI, 139–140
        versus H_2RA (histamine$_2$-receptor
            antagonists, 139, 140
    surgery,
        antireflux, 103, 140–141
        esohagomyotomy, long, 144
        laparoscopic Heller myotomy, 144
        myotomy, 144
        Nissen fundoplication, 140
        pneumatic balloon dilation, 143–144
    Tietze's syndrome, 44
    visceral hypersensitivity, 138
Tricyclic antidepressants (TCA), 44, 136,
        137, 138, 145, 151
TRPV1 (transient receptor potential
        vanilloid type 1), 66
Tuberculosis, 47
24-hour esophageal pH monitoring
    and diagnosis, 26, 27, 104
24-hour esophageal pH testing
    visceral hypersensitivity, 33

U

Ultrasonography
    gallstones, 46
    pneumothorax, 48
    Tietze's syndrome, 42
Ultrasonography, high-frequency
        intraluminal
    for esophageal motor events, 29–30

V

Ventilation perfusion scanning, 47
Ventricular hypertrophy, right, 50
Visceral hypersensitivity, 28
    acid exposure, 30–32
    and allodynia, 31–32
    autonomic function alteration, 33
    esophageal balloon distension, 28, 31, 34,
        60–62
    fMRI (functional magnetic resonance
        imaging), 33